DATE DUE

JUL - 4 1996	
MAR 3 1 1997	
UNBC 94 000981	
due Jan 6/99	
MAR 2 1 2000	

Troubled Bodies

Critical perspectives on postmodernism,

medical ethics, and the body

Edited by Paul A. Komesaroff

DUKE UNIVERSITY PRESS   *Durham and London 1995*

© 1995 Duke University Press
All rights reserved
Printed in the United States of America on
acid-free paper ∞
Typeset in Minion by Keystone Typesetting, Inc.
Library of Congress Cataloging-in-Publication Data appear
on the last printed page of this book.

Contents

Troubled Bodies

Introduction: postmodern medical ethics?

Paul A. Komesaroff

This is a book about medical ethics, albeit of a somewhat unfamiliar kind. It does not do what most books about medical ethics try to do: it does not attempt to identify general principles of good or right conduct as they might apply to medicine or medical research; it does not present a variety of ethical theories from among which a choice is to be made and propound one of them as the preferred option; it does not seek to provide criteria for determining the best action in a difficult clinical situation or to present arguments that are intended to resolve a specific ethical dilemma. It is not, in other words, concerned about "normative ethics"; but neither is it concerned with "metaethics," with the structures of ethical propositions and the ways in which they are used in ethical discussions.

The issues addressed in this book are both broader and narrower than these. They include the large-scale structure of the ethical dimension of medicine, encompassing the ethical presuppositions underlying the practice of healing and the theory of the body. At the same time, they encompass the reciprocal interdependence of medicine and the prevailing cultural structures. And they extend to the impact that medicine has had on the lifeworld—on that intimate and private realm of experience within which we live and construct realms of meaning and value.

In their various ways, the essays in this volume explore the conditions of ethics and the nature of ethical theorizing in relation to medicine. They address some of the ethical implications of new techniques and scientific insights—and, indeed, of well-established ones. They explore the medical construction of the body and its outcomes at the level of values. They thus cover a considerable variety of questions; they do so, moreover, from a variety of perspectives, with a variety of methods, and with a variety of conclusions. Accordingly, this work does not attempt to present a single, comprehensive critique of conventional medical ethics, much less seek to develop an alternative set of propositions to replace it. Its project is rather to raise issues and problems by drawing on the richness of contemporary theory and thereby, it is hoped, to help establish a ground for a proliferation of new approaches to these ancient problems.

Because the project of this book is somewhat heterodox, it may be useful to sketch some features of the cultural and philosophical context within which the need for such a series of reflections on medicine and ethics has emerged.

Ethics and medicine

I shall begin with some brief comments about the place of ethics in medicine. The ethical dimension of medicine manifests itself in widely differing ways. Some of these are obvious and have been extensively discussed. Medicine can contribute directly to the relief of suffering and pain. By overcoming or mitigating the effects of disease and physical disability that have hitherto been limiting and have compromised the range of available choices, it can help to release us from the limitations imposed by our biological facticity. Through innovations of knowledge and technique, important new questions can be raised for ethical consideration regarding our relationships with nature and with each other. At the level of face-to-face contact between patient and caregiver, a dialogue can be initiated which may enhance understanding of fundamental values and purposes and so expand our scope for informed and autonomous action.

Of course, in practice, the outcomes of medical knowledge and know-how are not unambiguously beneficent. Indeed, it has been argued trenchantly, by Ivan Illich and others, that the development of modern medicine has been associated with profoundly malign social consequences.[1] According to this view, medicine has been responsible for a degradation of intimate and meaning-endowing human experiences by transforming them into mere technical events. Rather than enhancing the knowledge and understanding of laypersons, these are actually diminished as a result of the transfer of decision-making power to a small group of often wealthy, usually socially conservative, and predominantly male individuals. It is Illich's view that medicine has actually produced a great increase in sickness and disease in modern societies—to such a degree that he is prepared to refer to the impact of contemporary medicine, in a famous oxymoron, as "one of the major epidemics of our times."[2]

To be sure, it is well-recognized that the practical applications of medicine are limited and distorted by social conditions, by the facts of poverty and wealth, of impotence and power. However, the argument is stronger than this. According to this view, expressed in vigorous debates extending over more than two decades, the adverse consequences of medicine are not merely the unintended effects of the application of an inherently benevolent set of techniques; rather, they are generated out of its underlying conceptions and its internal modes of organization. In spite of its own claims, it is argued, medicine leads inevitably to a loss of personal autonomy and to the contraction of the possibilities for action.[3] The sociologist Eliot Freidson states the moral issues directly:

> In essence, the process of treatment and care may be seen as a process which attempts to lead the patient to behave in the way considered appropriate to the illness which has been diagnosed, a process often called "management" by professionals. . . . Professional management generally functions to remove from the patient his identity as an adult, self-determining person, and to press him to serve the moral and social identity implied by the illness which is diagnosed.[4]

Even if the more extreme formulations of this aspect of the cultural critique of medicine are hotly disputed, it is obvious that not all of medicine's putative benefits are realized in practice. For our present purposes, however, what is of greatest interest from these debates is the underlying claim that the ethical component of medicine is of great breadth and scope. Ethical discourse, it is held, is not restricted to analyses of the principles that guide social policy on the one hand or the decision making of clinicians on the other. Medical ethics encompasses also the values that are presupposed by the technical apparatus and those that are generated by it, and it encompasses the social outcomes of medicine, as assessed in relation to their implications for the quality and meaning of everyday experiences, rather than just the consequences of specific acts. The essential insight here is that ethics is not merely adventitious with respect to medicine, affixed to it after the fact by philosophical experts. Ethics and medicine are intertwined; medicine, as Edmund Pellegrino once put it, is "a practice of ethics."

There are many trajectories along which medicine intervenes in society: these include the deployment of scarce material resources, the transformation of the world of individual experience, and the generation of new knowledge. All these cases are replete with ethical effects. With respect to the distribution of scarce resources, this is obvious. With respect to the implications for the social lifeworld, it is perhaps less immediately apparent but no less important; here, the ethical effects of medicine are generated by its own methodological imperatives. Where common social practices are formulated in the language of pathology, the possibility of a moral evaluation of them is introduced. Admittedly, it is not inevitable that moral judgments follow, for these depend also on local, variable cultural factors. For example, in at least the English-speaking Western societies, the treatment by medicine of alcoholism, homosexuality, and the so-called "eating disorders" both reflects and reinforces social attitudes to them and influences the ways in which they are dealt with at the level of the institutional structures.

The same process affects many other common experiences. The infiltration of the categories of medicine into the ways in which we think about pregnancy and childbirth, the menopause, sexual relationships, and caring for a sick relative, for example—or, for that matter, merely eating, exercising, or just lying in the sun—may profoundly transform the quality of these experiences. In these cases, medical modes of thought introduce into previously unproblematic life experiences evaluative criteria that are formulated in purposive-rational terms—that is, they are presented as purely technical values. However, the outcomes cannot be constrained within the technical discourse, and they spill over into moral-practical effects. The reason for this is straightforward: the medical reformulation of these experiences decisively affects the ways in which individuals can accommodate them at the level of meaning. They therefore also affect the ways in which individuals behave with respect to others. In part, too, this is because they do what they deny that they are doing: they incorporate an implicit vision regarding the good life, in the classical sense.

Not even at the epistemological level is medicine protected from ethical considerations. It is, of course, often enough observed that, in general, issues of fact and issues of value cannot be clearly separated from each other. With respect to medicine, this is particularly clear. Health and well-being are ethical values or, at least, are implicated in ethical theories in a fundamental way. Similarly, truth itself and the pursuit of knowledge themselves have well-defined ethical standings. At the same time, as we know from a half-century of investigations in the philosophy of science, what counts as truth in scientific theories is influenced by variables that are subject to social and historical determinations.[5] Both medicine and biological science—which lays claim to being the contemporary form of the theory of nature relevant to medicine—are inseparable from the epistemological and metaphysical assumptions on which they are based.[6] These assumptions, furthermore, which admittedly are installed at a deep level of the culture and are often not accessible to individual scientists, are themselves coupled to ethical perspectives. Indeed, as both Nietzsche and Heidegger pointed out in somewhat different ways, there are underlying ethical predispositions from which a whole culture cannot be dissociated: they form our traditions and our attitudes and "shape our historical being."[7]

Medicine and society, then, are interdependent. The technical outcomes of medicine and its conceptual forms may convey far-reaching social effects; conversely, the social forms find their expression in both medicine's theoretical structures and its practical techniques. Accordingly, medicine is not just an adjunct to the culture, a tool or an implement produced by it; rather, it itself contributes actively to cultural development and change. Much of cultural production is inextricably linked to values and moral-practical thinking; a fortiori, the same must apply to medicine. This is indeed the case: medicine is saturated with questions regarding ethical value, and these questions are at once constitutive of medicine and the complex outcomes of it.

To study the role of ethics in medicine, it is necessary to recognize that the ethical dimension is complex and multifaceted. From an ethical point of view, medicine serves a plurality of tasks. At least within the resources of the contemporary cultural conjuncture, there is therefore no single ethical perspective that can adequately capture the proper place of ethics in medicine, nor is there a single, unambiguous goal. Ethical reflections on medicine must seek to incorporate this diversity, as well as to accommodate the interdependence to which I have just referred between medicine and the cultural structures.

What is required, in other words, is a critique of society and ethics that is also a critique of medicine, and which both recognizes and promotes diversity. What is required is the fostering of critical reflections on medicine and its practices from a variety of perspectives and with a variety of theoretical styles. This approach—which this volume seeks to promote—represents a major departure from the usual way of discussing ethics in medicine or, for that matter, ethics in general. To appreciate the nature of the new departure involved and the specificity of what is proposed, it is necessary to return to the project of ethics and epistemology that has characterized the period of modernity.

Ethics in the age of modernity

Contemporary reflections on ethics in medicine derive in substantial part from the project in ethics which had its origins in the European Enlightenment around the mid-seventeenth century. The basic conviction that has guided this project has been the belief, inspired by science, that, in an unlimited, universal, and inexorable way, progress will occur toward greater knowledge and social and moral improvement; inherent in this vision, furthermore, is the confidence that this progress will be generated, and protected, by the application of reason.

The institution of this project presupposed a major reorganization in the processes leading to cultural production. This was not merely an abstract idea; the culture of modernity provided a structure and a mechanism for realizing this goal. As Max Weber first observed, and Jurgen Habermas has more recently elaborated, at the level of cognitive endeavor modernity was characterized by the differentiation of the substantive reason formerly expressed in religion and metaphysics into three relatively autonomous spheres: those of science, morality, and art.[8] The original impulse for this development was the disintegration of the unity of the erstwhile religious and metaphysical worldviews; however, it soon acquired an inherent dynamic of its own.

The older worldviews had provided unified ways of understanding based on common criteria. In the new one, separate regions of discourse and action were distinguished, each of which had its own specific task. Science, as it developed after the time of Galileo, gradually became the major intellectual practice devoted to the search for truth; ethics and jurisprudence assumed the role of carrying out the search for normative rightness, and art became the site for behavior directed toward eliciting and theorizing beauty; this last, somewhat later, gave rise to the academic discipline of aesthetics. Each of these areas was conducted by "experts," individuals with specific skills and knowledge whose activities were by and large restricted to one main field of activity.

In this new tradition of modernity, the object of theory became differentiated into the search for truth, for the good, and for the beautiful, three regions that were now rigorously distinguished as separate spheres of activity. These regions were distinct, but they were not completely independent. They were linked by their mutual dependence not on the totalizing force of religion, which increasingly became regarded as obsolete, but instead on the totalizing force of reason.

The possibilities and power of reason as it was conceived by the thinkers of the Enlightenment were unlimited. This reason was intended to be the tool that would render perspicuous the formerly obscure complexities of nature and society. Reason itself, however, was a complex cultural accomplishment with hidden presuppositions and profound implications.[9] For example, presupposed by the Enlightenment conception of reason was a particular notion of the subject. Reason was, after all, taken to be exercised by an isolated, monadic subject whose connection with society and embodied form were secondary characteristics and who, so it has been claimed, was "gendered" in the sense that it realized qualities strongly linked to "masculinity" while rigorously excluding others—such as passion, faith, and emotion—linked to "femininity."[10] The valuing subject had conferred on it a position and function similar to that of the knowing subject of modern epistemological theory. Both the ethical and the epistemological subjects took on a positivity that marked out a center in relation to which valuations and knowledge proceed. Values and knowledge have become viewed as properties possessed by a subject.

In each of the fields of science, morality, and art there was, as Taylor has put it, a tendency to "breathtaking systematization" and unification;[11] in the case of ethics and morality, the task was defined as the search for a rational justification of rules for good conduct. Indeed, morality itself became understood as a process of following rules, usually of universal application. This search for a single principle to guide action is a peculiar feature of modern moral philosophy. Older approaches to ethics and morality, which had previously commanded wide acceptance, such as the foundational role of the virtues or the recognition that there are a number of quasi-autonomous goods, were discounted.

In this "Archimedean view" of ethics, as Bernard Williams described it, ethical theories sought to justify themselves on the basis of a single philosophical method and general theories of human nature. Morality was given a very narrow focus; it was considered no more than a guide to obligatory action. Underlying assumptions differed, of course, from theory to theory; nonetheless, a common tendency was—once again, in the words of Charles Taylor—to

> unify the moral domain around a single consideration or basic reason, e.g., happiness or the categorical imperative, thus cramming the tremendous variety of moral considerations into a Procrustes bed. And there are other cramps as well. The notion that morality is exclusively concerned with obligations has had a restricting and distorting effect on our moral thinking and sensibility. . . . [I]t fails to cope with all that aspect of our moral thinking which concerns aspirations to perfection, heroism, supererogation, and the like. Once more, in Procrustes fashion, this is either assimilated to a foreign mould or rejected.[12]

The tendency toward unification was accompanied by a demand for a comprehensive systematization of moral theorizing. The two main contemporary examples of this are utilitarianism and Kantianism, which, in different ways, seek to organize everything around one basic reason. Both, furthermore, understand morality as a matter of formulating rationally based principles of obligatory action.[13] In the same way, the role of the philosopher is defined very narrowly. As with the great philosophical theorists of ethics, the philosopher's job is to identify a procedure or set of procedures that will generate good actions or propositions. In some theories, the possible contribution of the philosopher is even more limited—here we may mention Hare, for whom one of the main functions of the moral philosopher in relation to medicine was to clarify the use of "tricky terms" or the familiar passages from the early Wittgenstein, for whom the job of philosopher was to define a domain of meaningful language, which may well exclude moral discourse altogether.

This is not to claim that there have been no contrary tendencies in ethical theory since the Enlightenment. Quite the contrary, the project has been subjected to sustained, rigorous questioning. The philosophical interrogations of Kierkegaard, Nietzsche, Heidegger, and others, however, while they have raised doubts about the ethical project of modernity, have not supplanted it. Similarly, in modern ethics, and medical ethics in particular, various approaches exist outside the utilitarian and Kantian mainstreams of normative ethics; some of these draw on phenomenology, some on the Marxian tradition, some on a revival of the ideas of Aristotelian ethics.[14] These approaches form the basis and the inspiration for many of the essays in this book.

Problems with the project of modernity
and the postmodernist challenge

There can be no doubt that, viewed in terms of the sheer volume of its output, the culture of modernity—the project devoted toward securing objective science, universal morality and law, and autonomous art—was successful. However, this success was won at a price. The distance between the culture of the experts and that of the larger public grew. What accrued to culture through specializing treatments did not necessarily flow to the practices of everyday life. Indeed, the growing gulf between the categorial realm—the realm of theoretical constructions and systems integration—and the lifeworld of individual experience was argued by some, such as Husserl in his last, great work, to characterize the human condition in the age of modernity in a uniquely poignant and tragic way.[15]

The ethical project was deficient in several major respects. Excluded from the theorizing based on modern, systematic normative ethics, for instance, are many of the qualitative distinctions that used to be at the center of ethical theorizing. Visions of the good are neglected, as are discussions of the good life. As stated, the role of reason, in its hypostatized Enlightenment form, is taken for granted, and the possible foundational role of the virtues, or the fact of embodiment or sociality, is excluded from consideration as a matter of principle.

Of particular concern and importance is the narrow conception of freedom generated by this mode of theorizing. This is, in turn, due to the limited conception of the subject as isolated and individual, as separated from society and exempt from social constitution. As MacIntyre has pointed out, this series of assumptions represents one of the major weaknesses of the whole Enlightenment project. Indeed, he claims that it is seriously undermined by the lack of an adequate appreciation of the bond between ethical thinking and society. The modern or Enlightenment approach to ethics failed because it lost the bond, so important in premodern thought, between ethical thinking and society, between the individual and the polis.

The recognition of these deep problems inherent in the project of modernity has evoked many critical responses and proposed alternative strategies over the last two hundred years. The fundamental assumptions underlying each of the components of this project—that is, art, science, and morality—have been subjected to systematic scrutiny. One of the most interesting sets of responses has aroused particular interest in recent years: that often referred to under the general rubric of "postmodernism." Now, despite the fact that the term has been in use since the 1930s, the nature of postmodernism and its status as a concept remain extremely controversial. It certainly does not represent a unified theoretical school or movement; its role as an appropriate characterization of a historical period is doubtful, and its applicability as a tool of analysis for cultural phenomena in general is uncertain. It is understood in widely differing ways. For example, it has been referred to variously as a new historical epoch,[16] as a moment within the continuing cultural project of modernity[17] (that is, as a component either of modernity or of postmodernity), or, broadly, as a general cultural tendency or "cultural dominant" of late capitalism.[18] The specific details of this debate do not concern us here, although it is worth noting that one of the features often claimed to be specific for postmodernism—its recognition of reality as inherently paradoxical, ambiguous, and open-ended—was in fact a central feature of modernism itself, and so represents at least one respect in which postmodernism is a continuation of the latter rather than the result of a decisive rupture with it. In spite of these difficulties with the concept of postmodernism, in defined contexts the term remains a useful one, and it is possible to speak of some central tenets that would seem to be part of most contemporary accounts.

In general terms, postmodernism represents a response to the *aporia* of the project of modernity. Within it, the subject is granted a much more limited role, and the field of discourse is much more diverse and fragmented. Art, science, and morality are all understood to be much more heterogeneous than previously recognized, and the outcomes of a plurality of techniques and approaches. There is a rejection of the commitment to certain knowledge and the search for an irrefutable foundation for truth. There is a particular emphasis on the need for an ongoing reflection on, and awareness of, the process of the generation of cultural products, including, in particular, of knowledge.

Postmodernism declares the death of the "grand narrative," especially of the great cultural constructions of "humanity," of "the proletariat," of "womankind," of "beauty," of "truth," and of the project of universal "liberation."[19] It abolishes the central subject, from which truth and knowledge have flowed for three hundred years, and it abandons the notion of a single totalizing reason as the organon, guarantor, and guardian of knowledge.[20]

In the place of knowledge (in the singular), it erects discourses (in the plural),[21] which can proliferate, and may be incommensurable, but nonetheless are not excluded from the demands of rigor and complexity. In the place of reason, there are only "reasons."[22] In the place of the central, potent subject, it offers the "decentered" subject, no longer structurally disengaged from the social processes which constituted it, but implicated within them and constantly being generated by them. This subject is not a center within an abstracted space of epistemological, aesthetic, and ethical theory; it cannot be separated from the hermeneutical space of praxis and intersubjective communication, and, as we shall see presently, it cannot be understood apart from the irreducible and inexorable fact of its embodiment.

The postmodern world, then, is a place of infinite variety and diversity. In it there are no fixed, unchallengeable criteria for judgment. Instead, contending perspectives are fostered and encouraged. This world is a place of radical freedom, in which the existential choices extend not just to the external circumstances of one's life but to the nature of one's subjectivity itself. The postmodern person is not faced with a socially patterned telos to which he or she is subject, as had previously been the case. Instead, he or she has to choose—to choose radically, not merely the content or the direction of his or her life but the framework itself, the context of and the conditions for judgment. The postmodern person is thus *contingent*; this is, so it is claimed, the shared experience of the contemporary world.[23]

It should be added immediately that, in spite of these apparently radical commitments, the political implications of postmodernism remain controversial. For example, it is claimed by some that postmodernism excludes in principle the possibility of any coherent political theory,[24] and by others that it gives rise inevitably to a reactionary and antidemocratic politics.[25] On the other hand, it is also said to raise profound possibilities for political associations that are based not on old concepts such as "community" and "freedom," but on new ones such as "radical difference" and "openness to unassimilated otherness."[26]

In both its forms—as cultural critique and as putative political manifesto—postmodernism has been applied to art and art criticism and to other aspects of culture in the computer age. It may be said that it has been applied to a much more limited extent to ethical theory, and almost not at all to medical ethics. In a major work on postmodernism and art, Peter Bürger argues that contemporary art—which he characterizes as "post avant-garde art"—challenges many of the assumptions of modernism, in particular, the autonomy of art and the existence of well-defined aesthetic norms. Post avant-garde art is distinguished by a plurality of styles and tendencies; art as an institution still exists, but "the possibility of positing aesthetic norms as valid ones" does not. This reflects both on the artistic products and on aesthetic theory: for "(w)here the formal possibilities have become infinite, not only authentic creation but also its scholarly analysis become correspondingly difficult." All that is left from aesthetic theory is a "functional analysis" of the "social effects" of art works.[27]

The dissolution of aesthetic norms has meant a transformation in the nature of artistic creation. No longer is art subject to the category of beauty—which, as the principle guiding the production of artistic works, itself only came into existence with the Renaissance.[28] Instead, art can now subserve a wide variety of aesthetic interests, "an infinity of purposes," as Husserl said in another context. It can now challenge many of the distinctions formerly assumed to be inviolable—the distinction between art and everyday life, and between the high and the popular cultures, for example—and it can discover new tasks and experiment with new methods of creation.

While the explicit attention of the theorists of postmodernism to the questions of ethics and morality has been somewhat constrained, the potential relevance of this body of thought is evident. Ethics is concerned with a wide range of issues regarding values, the nature of the good life, and how one should behave in relation to other people both in general and in specific circumstances. Here, too, there has been a growing recognition that society is a battleground for contending value systems. As Max Weber—one of the great theorists of modernity—put it: "[F]orty years ago there existed a view that of the various possible points of view one was correct. Today, this is no longer the case; there is a patchwork of cultural values."[29]

Just as in the field of aesthetics there is no single category of beauty that can provide a universally applicable aesthetic norm, so also in ethics there is no longer a single, universally valid, category of the good. There is not one good, but an infinity of goods; there is not one method, but a multiplicity of discursive frameworks within which ethical analysis and debate can occur.[30] Once again, great systems are opposed rather than sought, and diversity is promoted and celebrated. The task of ethics is no longer to define the nature of the good, or duty, or "the ends of man," much less to derive irrefragable principles for correct action. Rather, it is to uncover the nature of ethical values and the process of value creation; it is to examine existing concepts and to expose their hidden assumptions; and it is to challenge the hegemony of existing value systems and so to expand the possibilities for ethical action.

Implications for medicine

There is a clear convergence between the cultural critique of medicine and the emerging understanding of the tasks of ethical discourse in the contemporary social context. This new conjuncture raises a number of questions regarding medicine and ethics which are taken up in various ways in the essays in this volume. These questions include the general problem of the interdependence of ethics and ethical discourse, and society; the question of the ethical implications of new medical technologies; related to these, the issue of the nature and status of the concept of personal autonomy; and the fundamental question regarding the role of the body in the production of ethical values. None of these is a new problem, of course; however, in the age of postmodernism (if such a locution can be employed) they are raised in new and forceful ways. Here, I shall mention a few of the issues at stake and then pass on to some general statements regarding the nature of ethical theorizing in medicine in light of these developments.

There have been many attempts to explicate the relationship between ethics and society; some of these are discussed in detail in the course of this volume. A representative argument to which I shall draw attention here, for both its suggestiveness and its difficulties, is that put forward by Alasdair MacIntyre, in his influential work, *After Virtue*. MacIntyre claims that "every moral philosophy has some particular sociology as its counterpart." All morality, he argues "is always to some degree tied to the socially local and particular"; therefore, "the aspirations of the morality of modernity to a universality freed from all particularity is an illusion."[31] Indeed, for him, the shaping of modern ethical discourse has been substantially determined by the specific cultural conditions established in the transition to modernity: he believes that in this transition the bond between the individual and the polis has been lost, as a result of which the old meaning of the virtues is no longer attainable. This is a general process:

> A living tradition . . . is an historically extended, socially embodied argument, and an argument precisely in part about the goods which constitute that tradition. . . . [T]he individual's search for his or her good is generally and characteristically conducted within a context defined by those traditions of which the individual's life is a part, and this is true both of those goods which are internal to practices and of the goods of a single life.[32]

MacIntyre's argument is suggestive, but it leaves open several important questions. It leaves open, for example, the question of the mechanisms by which processes at the level of society may be reflected in formulations at the level of theory; after all, these two realms would normally be regarded as incommensurable. It leaves open the question of the specific social variables that might be efficacious in this respect. It leaves open the questions about the nature of tradition and the historical variability of the process of interpretation.[33] And it leaves open the critical question of the relationship of the individual to society and the limits of individual decision making. These questions, as I have stressed, are not new; however, they are raised with particular urgency in the present context, in which the old certainties about the task of ethics, the nature of the subject, and the conceptual structure of medicine can no longer be taken for granted.

It may be mentioned in passing that on some of these questions MacIntyre himself has given different answers at different times. For example, while *After Virtue* closes with a wistful, somewhat resigned, call for the construction of new, local forms of community—a kind of modernized and differentiated polis or *Sittlichkeit* (understood in the Hegelian sense)—in an earlier essay, which addressed directly the question of medical ethics, he asserts that the new moral pluralism leads to the need for increased individual decision making in a narrower sense: "each patient has to be given the autonomy which will enable him or her to decide where he or she stands."[34]

But these are admittedly difficult questions. If the subject is "decentered"—if we can no longer conceive of ethical discourse and ethical decision making as radically disengaged from society—the old "thin" or "negative" concepts of autonomy and freedom need to be reconsidered.[35] There is, however, no single, clear alternative. Indeed, there is more than one postmodern formulation of autonomy, as several of the essays in this book make clear. Autonomy can be understood as the ability to engage in communicative processes unobstructed by either internal or external constraints; it can be understood as the capacity to choose the framework within which one's own actions will be judged; or, more generally, in the language of postmodernism, it can be understood as the process by which a discursively formed decentered subject enters the hermeneutical space of praxis together with other decentered subjects, similarly formed in discursive terms.[36] There are even more radical formulations. For Levinas, for instance, "ethics is the very origination of meaning" and autonomy, understood as similarly fundamental, is interpreted as an essential property of subjectivity as it arises in its immanent relationship to ethics. In this formulation, ethics and autonomy are inseparable at the originary level of being: "(s)ubjectivity is being subject to the other in an ethical relationship." These deep identifications emphasize the foundational role of language. Ethical reflection issues are always in an internal dialogue with language itself; there are no definitive formulations: we have only "the intrigue of language and ethics," an endless thinking back "from the Said to the Saying."[37]

The "object" of medicine is the human body. As Levinas has stressed, this body is deeply infused with questions relating to values. It is not, as earlier medical ideologies tried to portray it, simply an inert object of scientific knowledge or therapeutic action; it is both more complex and more elusive than this. The body is the source of meaning and meaning-creation; it is our internal horizon of knowledge and meaning; it is the perspective that we bring to bear on the world. These insights emerge in great and cogent detail especially from the work of Merleau-Ponty:

> "The body is the vehicle of being in the world, and having a body is, for a living creature, to be intervolved in a definite environment to identify oneself with certain projects and be continually committed to them. . . . [M]y body is the pivot of the world. . . . I am conscious of the world through the medium of my body."[38]

More recent theory has elaborated the interweaving of the body in the cultural world and the social and historical specificity of the meanings thereby produced. The body is a condition of medicine and ethics. It is, of course, the object of inquiry and the site of therapeutic action. That is obvious; what is less obvious is that it is itself discursively generated and therefore subject to social variables. The body is an effect of the extant, culturally contingent forms of discourse within which medicine operates and which also find expression in the contemporaneous political forms. Language and corporeality, therefore, are closely aligned:

> Constituted *in writing,* the discursive medium which governs the epoch and separates itself silently but efficiently from the spectacle, covering its own traces, the bourgeois subject substitutes for its corporeal body the rarefied body of the text. . . . The carnality of the body has been dissolved and dissipated until it can be reconstituted in writing at a distance from itself. . . . [T]he body is admitted only as a nameless momentum outside the real arena of meaning and endeavour, as an unruly mess of functions and afflictions which only in its object-aspect will discourse be able to name, categorise and subdue.[39]

As it is lived, the body is marked, inscribed, and made meaningful in relation to the culturally specific forms of intersubjectivity and language. The identity it acquires in this process is a gendered one, inscribed on the biological raw materials. Gender has particular significance with respect to the factors that shape the individual, for it carries a kind of internal generative force, with implications at the levels of knowledge, power, and ethics; it is also important to note that feminist thinkers—who embody the main contemporary forms of the cultural reflection on gender—have done much to bring together the experiences of the body and philosophy and social theory.[40]

Embodied experience generates meanings and values. Conversely, the limits of the body and its relations with others, and hence its boundaries and internal forms, are themselves the outcomes of ethical considerations. Both the body and ethics are social accomplishments; both are the effects of complexes of discursive systems. The autonomous body—the body as it stands in relation to the political culture—marks out a special trajectory in the manifold of social meanings and values.

In the age of postmodernity, medical ethics is a heterogeneous and differentiated subject. Within it, new problems are articulated and addressed, with new perspectives and new techniques. It arises from a deep skepticism regarding the old ideologies of both medicine and ethics; it remains particularly doubtful about the great systems that for more than two hundred years dominated the joint projects of ethics and modernity. Postmodern medical ethics rejects the conflation of ethics and normative ethics.

The three pillars of modernity—science, morality, and art—can no longer be kept radically separate. While they are each more diverse than they once were, their shared assumptions and their mutual interdependence are now evident. Within medicine, science and ethics—and, some would say, art—are indivisible. In spite of the fragmentation of worldviews, the proliferation of perspectives, a larger, more complex, unity perdures. There is a triad out of which both medicine and ethics are generated: the triad of the body, discourse, and society. It is one of the tasks of postmodern medical ethics to elucidate the elements and the interactions that characterize this triad.

The "fate of our times," as Max Weber said, is that fixed and final answers are no longer available to us: the world is "disenchanted"; the "ultimate and most sublime values" have retreated from public life.[41] Today, we must come to terms instead with fluidity and fragmentation, plurality and proliferation. This does not prevent us from asking the traditional global questions of value. Indeed, in relation to medicine, these questions are probably more pressing than ever. When we consider ethics and medicine, we need to consider what medicine is, what it does, and what it should be; at the same time, however, the same questions must be addressed to science and to society.

Conclusion

As I said at the outset, the essays in this book all seek to expand boundaries, to expose presuppositions, and to explore alternatives. They address some of the many facets of the relationship between medicine and values; in doing this, they explore various aspects of the body-discourse-society triad. Individually and together, they seek to reconstitute existing forms of discourse—including those derived from Marxism, feminism, poststructuralism, phenomenology, and conventional philosophical ethics—around the general problem of medicine and ethics.

The perspectives of the individual essays are diverse yet complementary. They draw on a wide variety of sources, from both within and without conventional medical ethics. The types of analysis employed are similarly diverse: there are studies of the broad structures of medicine, of its relationships with the social processes, of its techniques of knowledge and the character of the communicative processes it employs; and there are examinations of the internal character of the therapeutic relationship, of the nature and significance of embodiment, and of the impact of new medical technologies on the experience of the body. Some of the essays engage in a dialogue with bioethics; some question its underlying assumptions. Some examine the nature of medical knowledge; some focus on the clinical relationship and its particular problems. The treatments do not claim finality or completeness, and they certainly do not claim to provide a single perspective—regarded as 'postmodern' or otherwise—to replace the conventional ones. Indeed, today, such a quest is both impossible and inappropriate; our proper task is to do no more than to initiate and to suggest.

This book does not provide solutions for specific ethical dilemmas. It does not offer a general guide for right conduct. It offers a questioning, that is open and ongoing and which may lead to an enhanced appreciation of the depth and complexity of the dialectic of medicine and ethics. "The morality of thought," Theodor Adorno once wrote, "lies in a procedure that is neither entrenched nor detached, neither blind nor empty, neither atomistic nor consequential. . . . Nothing less is asked of the thinker today than to be at every moment both within things and outside them."[42] This reflection expresses both the contemporary conjuncture of our culture and the conditions for a deeper understanding of the nature and role of medicine. Only in this way might a reconciliation of medicine, culture, and everyday life become possible.

Notes

1   I. Illich, *Limits to Medicine* (London, Marion Boyars, 1976).

2   Ibid., p. 26.

3   See, e.g., J. Ehrenreich, ed., *The Cultural Crisis of Modern Medicine* (London, Monthly Review Press, 1978).

4   E. Freidson, *Profession of Medicine* (New York, Dodd Mead, 1970), pp. 329–330.

5   Cf. P. A. Komesaroff, *Objectivity, Science and Society* (London, Routledge, 1986).

6   M. Foucault, *Birth of the Clinic* (London, Tavistock, 1973); C. Canguillem, *The Normal and the Pathological* (New York, Zone Books, 1991); cf. M. Foucault, "The Politics of Health in the Eighteenth Century," in *Power/Knowledge: Selected Interviews and Other Writings, 1972–1977* (New York, Pantheon, 1980), pp. 166–182.

7   M. Heidegger, *An Introduction to Metaphysics* (New York, Doubleday, 1959), p. 13. See also F. Nietzsche, *The Gay Science* (New York, Vintage, 1974).

8   J. Habermas, "Questions and Counterquestions," in R. J. Bernstein, ed., *Habermas and Modernity* (London, Polity, 1985), pp. 192–216, and Habermas, *The Philosophical Discourse of Modernity* (Amherst, Mass., MIT Press, 1987), pp. 1–22.

9   M. Horkheimer and T. W. Adorno, *Dialectic of Enlightenment* (London, Allen Lane, 1973).

10   G. Lloyd, *The Man of Reason: "Male" and "Female" in Western Philosophy* (London, Methuen, 1984), and E. Grosz, *Sexual Subversions: Three French Feminists* (Sydney, Allen and Unwin, 1989).

11   C. Taylor, *Sources of the Self* (Cambridge, Mass., Harvard University Press, 1989), pp. 76–77.

12   Ibid., pp. 89–90.

13   Ibid., pp. 76ff.

14   In this context may be mentioned, among others, the works of Alasdair MacIntyre, Charles Taylor, Bernard Williams, Agnes Heller, Richard Zaner, and Hans Jonas.

15   E. Husserl, *The Crisis of European Science and Transcendental Phenomenology* (Evanston, Northwestern University Press, 1970).

16   J-F. Lyotard, *The Postmodern Condition: A Report on Knowledge* (Manchester, Manchester University Press, 1986), and J. Baudrillard, *Simulations* (New York, Semiotext(e), 1983).

17   A. Heller and F. Feher, *The Postmodern Political Condition* (London, Polity, 1988).

18   F. Jameson, "Postmodernism, or the Cultural Logic of Late Capitalism," *New Left Review* 146 (1984), pp. 53–93.

19   Lyotard, *Postmodern Condition,* pp. 31ff.

20   Ibid. See also J. Derrida, "The Ends of Man, " in *Margins of Philosophy* (Brighton, U.K., Harvester, 1982), pp. 109–136.

21   P. Murphy, "Postmodern Perspectives and Justice," *Thesis 11* 30 (1991), p. 118.

22   W. van Reijen and D. Veerman, "Interview with Jean-Francois Lyotard," *Theory, Culture and Society* 5(2–3): 277–311 (1988), p. 278.

23   A. Heller, "The Contingent Person and the Existential Choice," *The Philosophical Forum* 21(1–2) (fall–winter, 1989–1990), pp. 53–69. Agnes Heller refers to modernity here rather than to postmodernity; for the present discussion, however, the two may be regarded as essentially identical.

24   Jameson, "Postmodernism," p. 85–86, and S. Harding, "Feminism, Science and the Anti-Enlightenment Critiques," in L. Nicholson, ed., *Feminism/Postmodernism* (London, Routledge, 1990), pp. 84–87.

25   S. Benhabib, "Epistemologies of Postmodernism: A Rejoinder to Jean-François Lyotard," in Nicholson, *Feminism/Postmodernism,* pp. 107–130.

26   I. M. Young, "The Ideal of Community and the Politics of Difference," in Nicholson, Feminism/Postmodernism, pp. 300–323; also see Yeatman, "The Epistemological Politics of Postmodern Feminist Theorizing," *Social Semiotics* (forthcoming).

27   P. Bürger, *Theory of the Avant-Garde* (Manchester, Manchester University Press, 1984), 87, 122, 94, 87.

28   See A. Heller, *Renaissance Man* (New York, Schocken, 1981), pp. 252–253.

29   M. Weber, "The Meaning of 'Ethical Neutrality' in Sociology and Economics," in *The Methodology of the Social Sciences* (New York, Free Press, 1949), pp. 3–4.

30   Lyotard, *Postmodern Condition,* and Lyotard, *Just Gaming* (Minnneapolis, Minn., University of Minneapolis Press, 1985), pp. 50–59.

31   A. MacIntyre, *After Virtue,* (London, Duckworth, 1987), 225, 126–127.

32   Ibid., p. 22.

33   H. G. Gadamer, *Truth and Method* (New York, Seabury, 1975).

34 A. MacIntyre, "Patients as Agents," in S. F. Spicker and H. T. Engelhardt, eds., *Philosophical Medical Ethics: Its Nature and Significance* (Dordrecht, D. Reidel, 1977), pp. 197–212.

35 Cf. B. Williams, *Ethics and the Limits of Philosophy* (London, Fontana, 1985).

36 Cf. C. O. Schrag, *Communicative Practice and the Space of Subjectivity* (Bloomington, Indiana University Press, 1989), p. 201.

37 E. Levinas, *The Levinas Reader* (Oxford, Basil Blackwell, 1989), pp. 88–126, and Levinas, *Totality and Infinity: An Essay on Exteriority* (Pittsburgh, Penn., Duquesne University Press, 1969), pp. 72–77.

38 M. Merleau-Ponty, *Phenomenology of Perception* (London, RKP, 1962), p. 82.

39 F. Barker, *The Tremulous Private Body: Essays on Subjection* (London, Methuen, 1984), pp. 62–63, 66.

40 E. Gross, "Philosophy, Subjectivity and the Body: Kristeva and Irigaray," in C. Pateman and E. Gross, eds., *Feminist Challenges* (Allen and Unwin, 1986), pp. 135–143; see also J. Kristeva, *Desire in Language* (Oxford, Basil Blackwell, 1980) and L. Irigaray, *Speculum of the Other Woman* (Ithaca, N.Y., Cornell University Press, 1985).

41 M. Weber, *From Max Weber,* ed. H. Gerth and C.W. Mills (London, Routledge, 1948), p. 155.

42 T. W. Adorno, *Minima Moralia* (London, New Left Books, 1974), p. 74.

Divide and multiply: culture and politics in the new medical order

Doug White

To whom does one go if unwell? There is a wide choice close to where I live. There are a pharmacist, a newsagent, a firm of doctors, a bunch of assorted practitioners at the local sports medicine clinic, a community health center, several naturopaths, a chiropractor, a transcendental meditation center ("no worries," it advertises), and several psychologically trained therapists, and it is not very far to the nearest public hospital. No doubt this list could be added to, and anyone who lives in an Australian city almost certainly could access similar resources. Of course, there is a prior question before the one of "Where do I go?": How do I know I am unwell? Limitations on advertising by some practitioners means I am not as well advised here. According to locally prominent billboards, I'm not at my best if I get drunk or smoke or go outside without a hat, a shirt, and a slop of some greasy skin covering. Further advice comes from the magazines at the newsagency. While I haven't researched this area fully, I think it is quite possible that I am overweight, not well-tuned, and have skin and hair problems and that my sexual aura needs some attention. A woman would, I gather from what I have heard and read, be told of even more health problems.

There is something worth commenting on here. The enormous variety of healthmongers offers a great choice, and this is sometimes equated with a high degree of personal autonomy. No longer do I have to be satisfied with one form of medical practice, as was once the case, in a neatly graded hierarchy: specialist doctors, general practitioners, nurses, chemists. No longer do I have to enter the treatment area through one door, that of the general practitioner. The field is no longer quite so hierarchically structured, and certainly it is not governed by a single mode of theorizing; scientific medicine no longer is the only kind there is. That is how it seems. Yet the past wasn't quite as uniform as I have just presented it. I well remember a member of my family being taken to a faith healer many years ago, and there were all kinds of belief about of the efficacy of certain masseurs and other assorted cranks and quacks. The difference now is that the distinction between "true" medical practice and cranks or quacks is less clear. Nearly all the variety of practitioners now have been to some kind of school, and most have a certificate or diploma to prove it. The variety has probably become a bit greater, but the main difference is that all varieties are now certified. Looking at the customer rather than the provider, it might be considered that it is not an increased range of services that characterizes modern medical times, but increased gullibility. To be kinder, perhaps there is less confidence in any particular form of medical fixing.

Lack of confidence in any particular medical practice is not at all surprising. There are many pressures on us all that make it unclear as to whether we know we are sick or well. An inability to make friends with sexually preferred others might be indicative of unwellness, for which we should seek attention. Everybody gets spots or lumps on their bodies from time to time, but now it's a matter of a life-threatening warning, for who but an expert could tell us that it isn't breast cancer or incipient melanoma? Being a bit tired or irritable would most likely have once been put down to working too hard or having to put up with unpleasant social circumstances; now it might be just as well to see a psychotherapist or a naturopath. And so it goes on. In these circumstances, to which some people are immune, although the degree of resistance appears to be weakening, individual autonomy is rather more like anomie than a desirable state of independence. Uncertainty of meaning and definition is characteristic of both the providers and users of health services.

The great variety of services, and the intensity with which health advice is offered, is not at all in contradiction to an actuality of uniformity and hierarchy. The uniformity underlying the variety is that there is a technical solution to all problems. The intensity of advice, and the number of consumers of this advice, suggests that a great many people have come to believe that they no longer have to put up with any imperfect state. Anything from pimples to a vague feeling of not being treated quite right by the world has a solution. Since, of course, most problems have no solution, or no completely effective one, the opportunity for those offering solutions is endless. But the belief in technical solutions to human problems implies a belief in hierarchy; somewhere, out at the frontiers of science and engineering, a solution must exist. Hence the highest status is given to those with the superior technical skills—people such as brain surgeons, pharmaceutical producers, and genetic engineers (who have recently claimed that the ultimate problem of a limited life span can be overcome).

Autonomy and cultural diseases

If this sketch of the health and illness scene is broadly accepted, the ethical problem can no longer be regarded as one that applies exclusively to the practices of doctors and other medical professionals. Rather, it must now be recognized as a problem pervading our culture and society. The particular problems faced in medical encounters are real and specific, and they need to be resolved as they present themselves. But such resolutions are only partial and inadequate; the context in which such issues arise itself needs theorizing. For example, the question of whether or not euthanasia should be permitted is once again under debate as this article is being written. Nurses, it is reported, by a large majority favor the practice. Perhaps it is the ultimate in caring, somewhat consistent with a slogan I read recently on a young woman's T-shirt, "double suicide is the sublime culmination of love." Doctors, a little more careful of their claim to be the supreme life maintainers, have been more wary of public statements. Perhaps they are waiting for a code of "ethics" on the matter. The Right to Life organization has no doubts about the answer to the question: for them, euthanasia is murder. The issue would hardly arise outside of the context in which there is thought to be a technical solution to all issues. If it was accepted, generally, that people with intractable, terminal conditions must die, the technical issues would become subordinate ones: dying could be allowed, with support and compassion. But as technical means of maintaining existence have become so highly valued, we have no way except that of establishing rules for another set of technical procedures.

Those who possess the technical procedures stand in a hierarchically superior position. Caring, which of all human practices is among those most strongly typified by the reciprocity of loving one another, becomes polluted by the inequality of a power relation based on control of the techniques. The old codifications of religious dogma appear as cultural fossils when brought into relation with the culture that elevates the technical fix. The expectation of autonomy, of control over one's body, which is interpreted as the maximization of happiness, becomes converted into the passing of control to the person with the technical know-how. The question of euthanasia is not a particular question at all; that it is raised for public debate in the current manner is a symptom of a cultural disease, a cultural disease not addressed by those forms of practice which take a symptom as the disease itself.

But many medical encounters, it may be argued, are not at all characterized by the exertion of authority of technical knowledge. Medical dominance is an ideology of which many medical people are aware is held by others, but not themselves. Particularly in the more fashionable locations, like psychotherapy and at the community health centers, the practitioners may go to great lengths to avoid instruction and to avoid decision making. I believe this is not at all what it seems and will attempt to make my point through a couple of examples, one from personal experience and one I just made up. The first example is a dialogue with a doctor on a trivial matter:

> Me: I think I need glasses, at least for close-up work.
>
> Doctor: Why ask me, then? If you think you need glasses, you must need them. No one could know better than yourself.
>
> Me: Actually, what I want is a referral from you to a specialist who might tell me more.
>
> Doctor: If you want a referral, then I'll give you one. But I can't see what a specialist could tell you that you can't tell yourself.
>
> Me: Aren't there objective tests for farsightedness?
>
> Doctor: Yes, but it is up to you what you want to use your eyes for. To a jeweler or a watchmaker, farsightedness is a serious matter, but for some other people it doesn't matter at all. Do you read much?
>
> Me: Isn't it worthwhile, if I'm going to have trouble reading, which I do, I should get my eyes checked for other things?
>
> Doctor: O.K., I'll give you a letter for a specialist (which he recommended).

The encounter was pretty harmless. The doctor's authority was used in an attempt to enhance the autonomy of the customer; he might have thought he was engaged in an empowering dialogue. I suspect most people gain knowledge by being told something, but current ideas of autonomy inhibit people from using their authority directly. Authority has to pretend it doesn't exist. Imagine, though, a conversation of a similar structure:

> Customer (female): I think my nose is not well shaped.
>
> Doctor: Well, you know whether it is or not. It all depends on what you want to do with it. Noses are many different shapes, and none of them is perfect to everybody.
>
> Customer: I think I'd be more attractive to men if it were a bit better shaped.
>
> Doctor: That all depends on how you want to attract men, or whether you want to at all.

Customer: I'm sure I'm right. Anyway, that is what I want.

Doctor: Well, if that is what you want, I'll write you a letter of referral to a plastic surgeon.

In this conversation, the apparent autonomy of the client is recognized, but it is the weight of the cultural expectation that is actually at work. Doctors could scarcely be expected to act as a counterauthority, if they respect the wishes of those who come to them. But for a long period, this is exactly what doctors did do—that is, represent an authority which at times was in conflict with other authority. The doctor's only claim to authority here is as a voice of the technical solution.

But there are times when it is the case that medical authorities act against what are widely held beliefs. The campaigns against smoking tobacco provide one such example. Since the evidence here is quite overwhelming, there is obviously a case that people should be informed of it. There is a strong case that tobacco should be made unavailable, or permitted in limited quantities, to addicts. The campaign could be directed against the purveyors, as it is with heroin, and this is done to a degree in the case of advertising and sponsorship of sport. In times when authority took a different form, people were not *persuaded* to have immunization against diphtheria; it was compulsory. Now, the authority has to present itself as directed toward lifestyle, which puts it on the same ground as the advertisers of cigarettes. The campaign against lying unprotected in the sun takes a similar form. Certainly there is a need for public information; there is also good reason for action against the modes of production and consumption that damage the ozone layer. The authority, which presents itself as no authority, is that of preferred lifestyle, and this means its actions on the one hand are limited. On the other hand, it is unlimited, for there is no limit to preferred lifestyle; living is rather hazardous, and the method of exertion of authority even when there is an objective basis for it cannot be clearly distinguished from manipulative advertising or moral puritanism.

Medical dominance and the illusion of choice

To summarize the argument to this point: there are a very large number of forms of medical practice available currently. They come in three kinds: that which might be called nonprofessional, offered by magazines and the media generally; that which is certified (and it is a characteristic of our times that this certification area has largely replaced older forms of folk medicine, quackery, and so on); and that which is offered by state and quasi-state authorities, in which persuasion aimed at lifestyles has been added to those older forms of public health administration that bring us clean water, unadulterated milk, and mass immunizations. Beyond these directly medical or health practitioners and practices lie various forms of research, of which the highest points are in such things as genetic engineering and the manipulation of bodily chemicals. What all these have in common is the belief that the human body need have cures for disease, as well as remedies for what were once regarded as natural aspects of life and outside medical help, like personal appearance, difficulties in relationships, and so on. Medical practice has expanded beyond its old boundaries and has taken over areas that were the province of others, such as friends, relatives, and religious practitioners. It has been able to do this because of scientific and technical advances and because the dissolution of older forms of relationship between people has opened the way for the technical solution. The apparent great variety of medical practices is superficial and masks a great uniformity. Because what is masked is actually a transformation of the form of life, this transformation is scarcely at the level of conscious understanding and has not been theorized. Moral decisions in these circumstances are likely to be based on an ethical theory derived from earlier times, or on no theory at all.

Health practice was not always like this. The present situation is a relatively recent development. A good deal of thinking about medical practice has been devoted to demolition work on the old structure, and rather little to interpreting the nature of the new situation. Evan Willis in his book *Medical Dominance*, for example, gives good reasons for not accepting the once well-established hierarchy of health practice, in which medicine defined the legitimacy of others and gained control of the work of other health occupations.[1] Willis is rather less definite and critical about the forms of authority and power that have replaced it. To put this a bit differently, if new levels of practice develop, as has recently been the case in health care, what once existed seems old-fashioned, restrictive, and inhibiting; that which is new seems to be liberating of restriction and inhibition. For example, when the eminent Australian eye surgeon, the late Professor Fred Hollows, suggested that quarantining persons infected with HIV might be an effective way of controlling the spread of AIDS among Australian Aboriginal populations, he was saying something that is completely acceptable within what were once well-established modes of handling epidemics. Only recently, and perhaps still, people with any of a variety of common infections were forbidden to travel to Aboriginal "reserves." Today, although quarantine is still regarded as a legitimate instrument of public health policy, its use is almost completely restricted to the cases of a few exceptionally dangerous, highly infectious diseases. In the case of HIV, it is seen not only as scientifically unsustainable but also as socially objectionable. Indeed, the suggestion above made Hollows the subject of fiercely expressed criticism, those making the criticism against him often calling up images of biblical attitudes toward lepers, to separations of one lot of people from another, and to the formation of boundaries around groups of people.

A practice of quarantine, once consistent with epidemiological understandings and social practices, is no largely longer consistent with social attitudes. From the new level of thinking, it is abhorred. Professor Hollows's comments were not judged in relation to their "efficacy," but in terms of current values. Those with the new perspective seek to remake the whole of social life in their own terms, occasionally exhibiting the smugness and sanctimoniousness which they assume is the quality of those who hold older views. This dominance of the new occasionally creates difficulties for those who are absorbed into it. Not long ago, for example, a group of Muslim women in the Melbourne suburb of Brunswick asked for special time at the local swimming pool, time in which men were excluded. As Muslims, they did not want to expose their bodies to men in general. Currently popular belief implies that people should be able to do what they want, and perhaps should have these rights at the swimming pool. Currently popular belief says that people's autonomy is restricted if they adhere to ideologies and religious beliefs that put boundaries around them. The ethical principle that seems to be at work is that individual autonomy does not include a foundation in any belief, except that of universal individualism.

The dilemma here is characteristic of what is often called "postmodernism." The whole set of beliefs in individual autonomy, a set of relations between people based on the satisfaction of the individually felt needs of each one, is a postmodern condition. Health practices of the kind drawn attention to in the earlier part of this article are part and expression of that condition. Yet a search for universal ethical principle derives from an earlier time, a time when social principles were not regarded as the sum of individual desires. Confronted with this difficulty, one mode of handling the ethical problem is to turn it back on the person seeking attention or assistance, as in the dialogues included a few pages back. And, if it appears to the doctor that the client is actually subject to a directing morality, what should be engaged in is its removal, the promotion of empowerment or liberation. Truth can, in these conditions, only be technical;

knowledge can only be information when it applies beyond the individual; and wisdom is an obsolete category. Ethical questions are particular, appropriate to case studies, not capable of generalization. To this, it can be said that there is a general mode of thought at work, and we might ask, Who empowers the empowerers?

Cultural sources of modern medical practices

Medical practices, coming in the categories that we still recognize—as doctoring, nursing, and public health measures—are a product of modernism, largely of the nineteenth century. What we now know is a consequence of that period, and of its subversion. The medical practices of modernism grew out of earlier practices. The medical doctor replaced the person with the healing spirit, medical science replaced the spiritual and cultural values to which the groups of human beings adhered, and nursing as a professional division of labor partially replaced kinship obligations of caring. The changes were gradual, reaching their culmination in modernism—in societies which were much larger and whose members were joined together by communication systems of which the circulation of commodities occupied a central place, by common beliefs in nationalism, and by state authorities that controlled and administered the larger whole.

The trio of medical practice—doctors, nurses, and the administration of public health—which characterized health care in the nineteenth century and most of the twentieth century, did not cover *every* medical practice. It did, however, dominate the picture. More particularly, this trio represented not the universal character of that period but the health practices of the modernized states of Europe and North America. This is a crucial point which I shall elaborate.

My thesis is that the condition for the historical conjunction of doctoring, nursing, and public health was the formation of bounded and centralized nation states, which both could and needed to develop systems of health care. A medical system of this kind could only come into existence with the development of science, establishing principles of hygiene, an understanding of epidemiology, and laws of immunization. Some of these understandings came well before the nineteenth century, but they are characteristic nevertheless of the period of modernity, even if its precursors came as early as the time of the English Tudor monarchy and the English revolution. Doctoring may be seen in some senses as always dealing with abstractions, with the non-present or the invisible, at least since the shamans and tribal medicine-men, and of later Christian healers working with the mystically given spirit of healing.[2] The public societies of the nation-state, together with the development of scientific understanding, secularized doctoring. Its spiritual aspects became secular knowledge. Its delivery no longer required a shared belief of a spiritual or religious kind; it could be delivered to anyone.[3] Doctoring became a feature of a bounded state system, retaining the hierarchical position of a practice touched by the other world of spirit or God, but depending for this position on the basis of superior knowledge and protected technique. Its delivery was to a public or mass, made up of unknown people whose relation to the doctor was accompanied by a similar relation to that of others who occupied the same territory of the nation. The nation, as Benedict Anderson argues, is an "imagined community";[4] its members have a relationship with members of the nation with whom they have no direct relationship, that is unlike earlier societies based on known associations, often with kin relations.

A nation-state also has a central point of organization; it has a capital city, a bureaucratic governing point. A nation represented an accumulation of capital and had a requirement of a committed and effective workforce. A nation needed to articulate its significance in its own culture, literature, and language; a nation needed intellectuals.[5] A nation also engaged in defending its boundaries through war and diplomacy and in extending its influence—requiring again articulators and interpreters, patriotic citizens, and dutiful military personnel.[6] Doctoring existed before the modern, nation-state, period, but it was transformed within those times. Nursing as a profession, or a category within the division of public labor, did not. Nor did public health, even though attempts at such things did exist. (Well before public health as we know it existed, the English House of Lords made an early stand against air pollution; coal fires were prohibited during sittings of the House of Lords, so as not to offend the rural peers visiting London for their meetings.) Florence Nightingale did her pioneering efforts in establishing nursing as a kind of profession during the Crimean War. Public health regulations were established out of the necessities of maintaining the population of workers in moderately reasonable health.

Bismarck once remarked that one-third of the students of the great German universities of the nineteenth century died of poor health and malnutrition, one-third wasted their lives in dueling and dissipation, and the remaining one-third ruled Europe. The Germans permitted this wastefulness as a necessary condition of the formation of their intellectual stratum. A less permissive stance was taken toward those who attended the compulsory primary schools, the selective secondary schools, and the state teachers' colleges. Here discipline and the centrally fixed curriculum were intertwined. Prussia and later Germany showed the characteristics of a national system in a rather more full-blown way than the other states of Europe and North America, but others took the same direction.

The health professions and practices that existed until recently, and whose ideologies are still with us, were formed in this period. *Doctors* were and are trained in universities. Their practices are offered locally, but are derived from sources of knowledge beyond the confines of a specific locality. Though registered and licensed by national bodies, the knowledge that lies behind their practices is formed by a larger process which transcends national boundaries, that of science.[7] Pasteur is celebrated in France as a citizen of that nation, but his national home is irrelevant as far as his discoveries are concerned. Doctoring, throughout the period of the dominance of the nation-state, although necessary to that nation could not be controlled by it. In the formation of the modern doctor, the universality of the healing spirit became replaced by the universality of scientific medicine: doctors claimed their own ethic. It remained beyond the control of the locals, but in a manner different from that of the past, its acceptance depended on its efficacy, not on shared belief.[8]

Nursing followed a different path. It moved from something done for others who had a particular relationship with the person needing care, to a requirement of a national system. Nursing became a function of the society rather than a kinship role, or something carried on by local, known people. Nursing, that is, delivered caring to unknown others, although those who received care could still expect it to have personal qualities. In many countries, vestiges of the older mode of nursing still exist, as when a family with a member in the hospital will arrange for someone to do the nursing. But public health, particularly that related to the military forces, which a modern nation required, meant that nursing became state sponsored. Nursing moved from the family to the nation. Its abstraction from the family situation did not mean it gained mystery, merely a wage. It developed a subordination to doctoring. It did not share in the abstract world of science, but did joint doctoring in the abstract world of the commodity form. Nevertheless, nursing remained tangible and understandable; like being a parent, there was a time when it did not seem beyond the possibility of anyone, or at least any woman.[9] Nursing was hardly a profession.

The third element of the health system of modernity, *public health*, depended on the combination of scientific understanding and a state authority with control over the population. That control required the acceptance and to a degree participation of the people, just as did the other great systems of modernity, the schools and the law. A set of enforcement agencies existed, but these served largely to administer and in the margins to impose penalties. Public health had compulsory aspects to it, but was also an area of popular demand.[10] The existence of such a system could scarcely be a possibility without the popular acceptance of the nation and its state.

The dissolution of the old order

In these conditions, a health ethic of a certain kind developed. A dual hierarchy, of state and doctors, existed. The authority was for the most part accepted. The population, though divided economically, was part of one nation. An expectation of behavior toward others with much in common existed. The conditions of life were more or less given, and expectations of what was to be got out of life were those of a relatively stable existence.

Medical practice, along with other practices, now occurs within a quite different context. Anthony Giddens paraphrases the position of Jean-François Lyotard, the author most responsible for popularizing the notion of postmodernity:

> Postmodernity refers to a shift away from attempts to ground epistemology and from faith in humanly engineered progress. The condition of postmodernity is distinguished by an evaporating of the "grand narrative"—the overarching "story line" by means of which we are placed in history as beings have a definite past and a predictable future. The postmodern outlook sees a plurality of heterogeneous claims to knowledge, in which science does not have a privileged place.[11]

Giddens does not accept Lyotard's view. A postmodern order does exist, or will come to exist. It is modernism that swept away all traditional types of order. The changes brought about by modernism are profound: "On the extensional plane they have served to establish forms of social interconnection which span the globe; in intensional terms they have come to alter some of the most intimate and personal features of our day-to-day existence."[12] Postmodernism for Giddens is modernism brought to its fullness. Whether we have one discontinuity—from "traditional" to "modern"—or two, including from "modern" to "postmodern," is an argument that will not be settled for some time. For our purposes it doesn't matter very much. The society of modern times certainly constituted a break from previous periods, but it did create in science and other forms of theory an authority, and it did create in the nation-state a bounded entity. Taken together, these offered a temporary (in historical terms) stability, although a stability characterized by economic and industrial progress, and in that sense a continuing progress. John Hinkson,[13] in his analysis of Lyotard's *Postmodern Condition* largely accepts Lyotard's observation, but contends that something like a grand narrative exists in the universal interchange of information and commodities. It is this, which begins with modernism, which has weakened the boundaries between nations and dissolved the old national authorities. The development of productive forces has been enhanced by the incorporation of intellect into its technology, a process described by economists under the heading human capital. The science produced by the great theorists of modernism—the science of Newton, Lyell, and Darwin—was largely interpretive: it gave an explanatory order to the world that broke from the religious explanations of earlier times. From about the beginning of the twentieth century, with the discovery of radioactivity, the rediscovery of Mendel's work on genetic transmission, and the speculations of Einstein on the relation between mass and energy, science began to penetrate and change reality, as well as offer interpretations. From this time theoretical science gradually lost its outside-of-nature interpretative preeminence and became a source of technical innovations. Since the 1950s the vast expansion of intellectually skilled people gathered momentum, a momentum which it still has, and the universities, the centers of enlightenment of modern times, became increasingly the center for the development of technical manipulation, of the material and the social world.[14]

To put it simply, by way of a summary of these somewhat provisional arguments, the condition that is sometimes described as postmodernism is characterized by three things: (i) the adoption of theoretical forms that offer release from the limitations of the given—that, for example, deal with the genotypes of bodily existence rather than the phenotypes of experience; (ii) a tendency to analyze and describe phenomena in terms that have vacated the ground of explanation and hence offer no generalized picture of the world; and (iii) the rise of a social stratum, the intellectually trained, which carry these new forms of practice to all the corners of existence. On the one hand, freedom from all constraints—of moral authority, of nation, of cultural capital, of patriarchy, of disease, of limited life span—is promised and celebrated in seemingly endless attempts to deconstruct and deauthorize the old givers. On the other, each person is left individually to expect and demand what is promised.

In these conditions, when much is promised, the old medical order cannot maintain itself. The old order was constituted around three levels of practice.[15] Let's look at them from the "top" down, from the highest level of abstraction to that which involved the most direct relationships. Doctoring, medical science, was founded on a universalized science and rationality, derived from the scientific branches of the Enlightenment, from an approach opened up by Newton and later followed by the great systematizers of biology—Darwin, Pasteur, Koch, and numerous others. The relationships between scientists, relationships that occurred in an extended form through the printed word of the book and the scientific journal, produced the knowledge upon which scientific medicine could develop, but of course the world within which this knowledge was created was not one in which patients lived. It was a world of scientific discourse that was abstract and infinite in its hopes of achievement, but bounded, in that its activities were defined differently from those of national or everyday life. It was drawn upon, rather than the maker of people's lives. The nation provided another level of practice, and this was regulated by the nation-state. Here doctoring was licensed and regulated, public health measures were authorized, and abstract nursing-care was established. Public hospitals were built. The ill— the patients and clients of medical practice—in some part at least inhabited the same area as the practitioners. Popular demands and social engineering of the Fabian socialist kind could both be effective here: on the one hand, an expectation that the nation was that of the people who could make demands on it; on the other, that social engineering made possible by the existence of the state could be effective. At another level again, health practices of a local kind, based on family and community also existed. Here people looked after one another, mothers applied ointments and lotions to their children, and local healers who on another level could be called cranks and quacks flourished.

The condition called postmodernity is an indication of the destruction of or severe damage to this world that once seemed so stable. Looking back on it, its structuration can be seen as intrinsically unstable. The nation held together the universal and abstract, and the local, direct, and concrete in a manner that could not last. For while establishing a bounded life, and drawing on sentiments of belonging that had previously been the province of ethnic groups in creating nationalism, the nation was also a center of national capital. Capitalism, as we have often had explained to us, is progressive—continually revolutionizing its techniques of production and extending its market. As a result, the nation erodes its own boundaries. That has been a tendency since the beginning of capitalism, as Marx and Engels pointed out with such rhetorical skill in the

Manifesto of the Communist Party. What is new is the drawing in of science with production, the use of the underlying structures of the atom, the gene, and the depths of our psyches in production and advertising. What was the independent area of rational science becomes a resource for production; what were human talents and human labor become another resource, human capital; and what is offered to all who once found meaning and purpose in some combination of universality, nation-belonging, and close relations are the market and the commodity.

Implications for health practices

In this collapsed and yet highly energetic state, a kind of social "black hole," what happens to medical practice? The doctor becomes trained in techniques, including the techniques of patient and "community" management, and authority rests only on expertise, an expertise about which only judgments based on the fulfilment of personally felt needs can be made, and of these there is no end. The nurse, now schooled in the academy, one of the intellectually trained, gains professional status by control of the technical equipment. Hundreds of practitioners offering bodily and psychological techniques flourish. The public health authorities, armed with analyses that show that lifestyles can be hazardous, move into their manipulation, enjoining us to run along footpaths, remember what it was like to be drunk, eat less salt, and boil water in stainless steel kettles. In those conditions a general ethic of medical practice is difficult to establish, for upon what would it be founded? The ethical question becomes one of the best use of technique in each case, and collapses into the kind of legal tussle characteristic of disputes over backyard fences.

Criticisms of this situation in health practice, or anywhere else, can be made, and often are, on the grounds of a preference for an older order of authority. Such criticisms do not have much significance, for they usually are expressions of a personal preference or regret: the editors of *Quadrant* and *Commentary* regret that there is no moral authority in the world, just as some clergymen wish that women did not want to be priests. But the old moral orders have adjusted their faith and diluted their substance to the point of emptiness in an effort to keep up their clientele; as Gellner says of modernist Christian theology, its elusive content asymptotically approaches zero. Freedom from directing authority and guilt-producing dogmas can scarcely be regarded as something to organize politically about. Individual responsibility is something to be valued, to the degree that it actually exists. Nevertheless, some basis for a way out of the emptiness of general values is necessary, for a condition that offers limitless satisfaction of unlimited needs is as unsustainable as a continually exploited natural environment. It makes the health hill too large, it offers eternal anguish about health, and it provides no basis for the individual responsibility that is said to be its foundation.

Where can a basis for such a way out be found? Possible strategies can be identified at a number of different levels. One potential point of entry into the field is to consider the actually existing characteristics of our bodies—that is, to put back into the center of consideration our nature. Fiona Mackie, in a comment on Germaine Greer's book *The Change: Women, Aging and the Menopause,* writes appreciatively of Greer's contribution "toward our regaining of this experience in our own terms."[16] Greer, rather than regretting becoming older, celebrates the new understandings of her body, reunites the "emphasis on spirit with a new rootedness within the body." If such an approach were generalized and talked about, autonomy might come to have a fuller meaning—a recognition of limits, boundaries, and inevitability. But this always carries with it the possibility of narcissism unless it is accompanied by newly developed forms of association, including community. Again, this does not need invention, but the drawing of attention to possibilities within present realities.

In the development of the nation, other forms of relationship such as the family and those of the locality and the ethnic associations between people with a common history were subordinated. With the development of internationally extended relationships the nation now is shifting into history. We do not, however, have to follow the path of progress of modernity and postmodernity in such a one-sided fashion. Certainly we may welcome the demise of "rural idiocy" that the restricted life of the village offered and welcome the end of national chauvinism that went along with the nation as a dominant social form. But the possibility of valuing, in their different ways, all these forms of association is also on the agenda (as they say in management ideology). It is not just a theoretical possibility, but one that is being worked out in the revival of ethnic association throughout the world.

To return to the opening paragraph of this essay—the discussion of the diverse range of contemporary health practices—the variety itself is seen, on one level at least, as a question of choice, and it is vigorously defended by many consumers for this reason. On the other hand, many practitioners are less sanguine about the deregulation of privileged position and lay claim to some degree of social or legal protection. Now it is quite plausible that each perspective has, in its own way, some validity—that is, that there are plausible arguments in support of the position that a large number of health practices work quite well, and, at the same time, that a particular practice should not be accepted merely on the basis of claims arising from that practice alone. To resolve these two apparently conflicting positions, and to answer the question about who licenses and limits the activities of individual practitioners, it is necessary to resolve the contradiction between two widely held value positions. On the one hand, there is the belief that everybody should have the right to choose what suits him or her and should therefore enjoy unlimited access to all possible services. On the other is the view that people should not be subjected to false claims and misleading advertising and that there needs to be an authority which ensures that such excesses do not occur. In the abstract, this problem is not at all easy to overcome, because in the current social context the old authorities—represented by such bodies as the Vatican, the Central Committee of the Communist Party, and the authority of the nation-state's public health system—no longer command widespread legitimacy.

Fortunately, in practice, the problem is often much less difficult. There are large areas where empirical evidence can be decisive. The facts on, for example, tobacco are well known: while it is widely agreed that tobacco would not, or could not, be prohibited from sale, it is also accepted that people should be informed of its dangers, that false advertising (which is pretty well all advertising) should be prohibited, and that nonsmokers should not be subjected to that practice in which they have decided not to take part. These principles could be extended. If chiropractors make false claims for the consequences of spinal manipulation that should not be allowed either, but nor should these practices be banned. And so on. Such an approach would require the existence of a state body with a defined area of authority to scrutinize the scientific evidence, and this raises questions of its own. A few things about it can be said directly—for example, that it should not be composed of members of any single branch of medical practitioners, and that whatever it says should be open for contestations; however, many potential (and most likely, intractable) problems remain.

In particular, there would be many matters on which this kind of rational authority would not be able to adjudicate. The most obvious of these are matters of morality. Certainly, discussions of moral issues are at least as important for the process of making judgments about medical practices as are discussions about scientific matters. However, it is both difficult and dangerous to establish a state body as a moral authority. This is because moral discourse should most sensibly be a discussion of the ways in which we want or ought to live our social lives in the local contexts of our particular forms of life and our particular communities. Attempts to develop institutions that deal with moral issues at the systemic level invariably obstruct such deliberations. This does not only apply to medicine. In government and economy, to take a parallel case, we are given lessons in economic rationalism by politicians and treasury officials; it would, however, be more appropriate for us to be given information about the rational use of resources, labor, and trade and to proceed to discuss this in a context of the forms of productive life we should need and value.

The problem of deciding about the most appropriate and desirable forms of medical practice, then, is not likely to be solved either by simple choice or by the exercise of state authority in the modernist sense; nor is it likely to be solved by backward-looking claimants for moral authority, whether as neo-Papacy, neo-Stalinism, or neo-Leavisite. There seems to be no alternative but to put our hopes in an informed public—informed both morally and empirically. However, that "informed public" is itself a multifaceted entity in a continuous process of formation and fragmentation. Accordingly, any attempt at a solution along these lines merely raises new, still more difficult, theoretical problems.

This may seem an unsatisfactory note on which to end. However, it does point to directions in which more work of both a practical and a theoretical nature needs to be done. For better or worse, the old medical order has gone and cannot be revived. The suzerainty of universal scientific medicine is an obsolete phase. What has taken its place is uncertain and equivocal: that which parades as choice is often a narrowing of choice, and that which claims to fill the moral vacuum is often just as empty. Nonetheless, out of the complex and variegated ensemble of practices that has come to characterize health care, new possibilities arise, along with unprecedented opportunities within social groups for the building of cultural meaning and significance.[17] Whether these opportunities will be realized, and what they will mean for medicine, we can only wait and see.

Notes

1   Evan Willis, *Medical Dominance* (Sydney, Allen and Unwin, 1983).

2   Mircea Eliade, *Shamanism: Archaic Techniques of Ectstasy* (New York, Bollingen, 1966).

3   Cf. Erwin H. Ackerknecht, *A Short History of Medicine* (Baltimore, Johns Hopkins University Press, 1983).

4   Benedict Anderson, *Imagined Communities* (London, Verso, 1983).

5   Geoff Sharp, "Constitutive Abstraction and Social Practice," *Arena* 70 (1985), pp. 48–82.

6   See Anderson, *Imagined Communities*; see also Perry Anderson, *Lineages of the Absolutist State* (London, New Left Books, 1974).

7   See Willis, *Medical Dominance*, esp. chapter 4.

8   Cf., however, Michel Foucault, *The Birth of the Clinic* (London, Tavistock, 1973), chs. 3 and 4.

9   See B. Abel-Smith, *A History of the Nursing Profession* (London, Heinemann, 1960), and V. L. Bullough and B. Bullough, *The Emergence of Modern Nursing* (London, Macmillan, 1969).

10 See e.g. F. Cartwright, *A Social History of Medicine* (London, Longman, 1977), and R. H. Shryock, *The Development of Modern Medicine—An Interpretation of the Social and Scientific Factors Involved* (Madison, University of Wisconsin Press, 1979).

11 Anthony Giddens, *The Consequences of Modernity* (Cambridge, Polity, 1989) p. 2.

12 Ibid.

13 John Hinkson, "Post-Lyotard: A Critique of the Information Society," *Arena* 80 (1987), pp. 123–155.

14 See J. R. Ravetz, *Scientific Knowledge and Its Social Problems* (Middlesex, Penguin, 1971), and Howard L. Kaye, *The Social Meaning of Modern Biology* (New Haven, Conn., Yale University Press, 1986).

15 The argument developed here draws heavily on Sharp, *Constitutive Abstraction*.

16 Fiona Mackie, "The Hidden Ones: The Despotic Politics of Menopause," *Arena* 98 (1992), pp. 15–22.

17 Doug White and Paul James, "The State of Modernity in Transition," *Arena* 98 (1992), pp. 5–9.

Abortion and embodiment

Catriona Mackenzie

Feminist perspectives on abortion focus on a fact the moral implications of which are either overlooked or considered unimportant by most other disputants in the debate. This is the fact that a fetus is not a free-floating entity about whom questions of potentiality and personhood arise as though in a vacuum. Rather a fetus is a being whose existence and welfare are biologically and morally inseparable from the woman in whose body it develops. From a feminist perspective the central moral subjects of the abortion question are thus not only, or not primarily, fetuses but women.

Within an influential strand of the feminist philosophical literature it has been usual to understand the moral dilemmas arising from this unique relationship between a fetus and a woman in terms of a conflict of rights and to defend a woman's right to abortion via the notion of bodily autonomy. In its crudest form, the alleged conflict is between (a) the "right to life" of the fetus, a right based on the presumption that it is a being deserving of some moral consideration, and (b) the right of the woman to bodily autonomy, that is, her right to decide what happens in and to her body. In attempting to resolve this conflict in women's favor, feminist defenders of abortion have taken two main lines of argument.

The first, articulated best by Mary Anne Warren, argues that in abortion decisions the woman's right to bodily autonomy must always prevail over any rights which may be claimed on behalf of the fetus.[1] This is because the only beings with full moral standing are persons. Not only are fetuses not persons, they are not even personlike enough to warrant our regarding them as if they were persons. Indeed, Warren claims that an eight-month fetus is no more personlike than the average fish. On this view, then, the "right to life" of the fetus, to the extent that it has such a right, cannot possibly outweigh the right of a person to one of the fundamental rights of persons: the right to bodily autonomy. In fact, Warren claims that having an abortion is morally equivalent to cutting one's hair.

The second line of argument is best represented by Judith Jarvis Thomson and, following her, Christine Overall.[2] Their claim involves a sophisticated reinterpretation of the claim that even if a fetus does have a right to life, the woman's right to bodily autonomy overrides that right. By trying to show that even if the fetus is a being with moral standing it has no automatic right to occupancy of a woman's womb, their argument seeks to undermine the basic premise of the conservative position on abortion—namely, the premise that if fetuses are persons, that is, beings with full moral rights, then abortion is necessarily wrong.

My aim in this article is to defend a feminist perspective on abortion by showing that questions of women's autonomy lie at the heart of the abortion issue. I shall argue, however, that the conflict-of-rights framework and rights-based models of bodily autonomy are liable seriously to misrepresent both the nature of abortion decisions and the reasons why the availability of abortion is essential to women's autonomy. My dissatisfaction with this kind of approach centers on four related concerns. First, a conflict-of-rights approach fails adequately to address the issue of responsibility in pregnancy and abortion. Hence it mischaracterizes both the nature of the moral relationship between woman and fetus and the kind of autonomy that is exercised in pregnancy and abortion. Second, it tends to oversimplify our conception of the status of the fetus. Third, it leads to a misconstrual of the notion of bodily autonomy because it is inattentive to the kind of reflective bodily perspective that arises from a phenomenological account of pregnant embodiment. Finally, defending abortion solely on the grounds of women's right to bodily autonomy logically requires that the right to abortion cannot entail a right to secure the death of the fetus but only a right to fetal evacuation.

I shall argue that a strong feminist case for abortion needs to construe a woman's right to obtain an abortion as the right of an autonomous moral agent to be able to make a decision about whether she wishes to take responsibility for the future well-being of a being dependent upon her. In choosing an abortion, in other words, a woman is not merely choosing not to allow the fetus occupancy of her uterus. Nor is she merely choosing not to undertake responsibility for a particular future child. Rather, as Steven Ross has pointed out, she is choosing that there be *no being at all* in relation to whom she is in a situation of such responsibility.[3] To require that a woman has no right to secure the death of the fetus, at least in the early stages of pregnancy, thus violates her autonomy.

Now against this claim it could be argued that here the woman is not only making decisions about her own life but about that of another. What entitles her to make such a decision? The next three sections of the article attempt to answer this question. In the second section I make some suggestions as to how we should understand the notions of responsibility and autonomy in pregnancy, while the third section assesses the moral status of the fetus both from the point of view of its intrinsic moral properties and from the point of view of its relationship with the woman in whose body it develops. Building on the previous two sections, the final section draws on a phenomenological account of pregnancy in order to explain the connection between autonomy, bodily autonomy, and pregnant embodiment. My criticisms of the rights-based accounts of bodily autonomy emerge from this discussion.

Responsibility and autonomy

Appeals to responsibility in the context of the abortion debate usually trade on the asymmetry between the situation of men and women with regard to pregnancy. The asymmetry is that while it is always possible for men to evade or even remain blissfully unaware of the consequences of their actions where those actions result in pregnancy, the same is not true for women. Further, it is women alone who are physically able to sustain the fetus. Thus women come to be held "responsible" for what was after all a joint action. Given this context, it is hardly surprising that feminist defenses of abortion often attempt to shift discussions of the abortion issue away from the question of responsibility. Thorny as it may be, however, one of my central claims is that the issue of responsibility is crucial for an understanding of women's moral autonomy with respect to pregnancy and abortion. In this section I attempt to outline an adequate feminist approach to the question of responsibility in pregnancy and abortion.

A number of different aspects of responsibility are often conflated in the abortion debate. To disentangle these I want first to distinguish *causal responsibility* from *moral responsibility*. By causal responsibility I mean simply responsibility for the direct causal consequences of one's actions in cases where those consequences can be said to be reasonably foreseeable and where a person's actions were freely chosen. In this sense, a woman can be said to be responsible for the existence of the fetus in much the same way as she can be said to be responsible for getting drunk, in that it is *her* actions, in this case along with those of another, which have brought about this outcome.[4] Although conservatives do not usually make an explicit distinction between causal and moral responsibility, the conservative claim seems to be that in the case of pregnancy, because the outcome here is to have brought into existence a being with full moral standing, then a woman's *causal* responsibility necessarily entails a *moral* responsibility toward maintaining the existence of the fetus.[5]

Feminists and liberals have responded to this claim in a number of ways. The approach of Warren and Tooley, for example, is to attempt to shift the focus of the abortion debate away from questions of moral responsibility and toward a consideration of the actual present status of the fetus with respect to personhood. Their argument is that because fetuses are not persons and therefore do not have rights, abortion is morally permissible.[6] A second approach aims to show that one does not necessarily have automatic moral responsibility to maintain the existence of a being dependent on oneself, even if that being does have full moral standing and hence a right to life. This is Thomson's approach in the examples of the violinist and Henry Fonda.[7] As Warren and Feinberg have shown, however, this strategy fails because the examples chosen are disanalogous to the case of the fetus in one relevant respect, namely with respect to causal responsibility.[8] The strategy thus begs the question. Yet another tactic is to claim that the attribution of causal responsibility is a lot less straightforward than it might appear and thus to argue that causal responsibility for the existence of a being does not necessarily mean that one is required to assume moral responsibility for maintaining its existence. For to what extent is a person still morally responsible for the consequences of an action if they have taken reasonable precautions against those consequences occurring? Thomson's example of the houseowner covering her windows in wire mesh to prevent the entry of people-seeds seeks to undermine in this way any necessary connection between causal and moral responsibility.[9]

While these responses have been partially successful in exposing some of the assumptions at work behind the seeming self-evidence of the conservative argument, they nevertheless fail adequately to come to terms with the question of moral responsibility in pregnancy because they concede too much at the outset to the conservative notion of moral responsibility. This is particularly true of the last approach which forces Thomson, after a series of increasingly bizarre examples, to attempt to dissolve the question of responsibility by an appeal to decency.[10] What needs to be pointed out is that the conservative account of moral responsibility is premised on a set of assumptions that are fundamentally oppressive to women, for it is significant that in this whole debate about responsibility there seem to be only two possible ways for women to get pregnant: either they are raped, in which case they have no causal responsibility for the existence of the fetus although according to some conservatives they nevertheless have a moral responsibility toward it, or they are not raped, in which case they are held to be fully responsible, in both a causal and moral sense. In neither case, however, is men's moral responsibility ever seriously discussed, despite their obvious causal involvement in the pregnancy. The consequence of this blindness is that moral responsibility in pregnancy gets construed extremely narrowly, as just responsibility toward the fetus, and in a way that seems to commit women to maternity.

The challenge then seems to be to envision a notion of moral responsibility in pregnancy that acknowledges the moral complexities of the situation and of the decision facing a woman who is weighing the choices of abortion or maternity, but that does not imply that the only possible morally responsible course of action is to choose maternity. My starting point here is to accept, without argument at this stage, both that the fetus does have some moral significance and that this is in part why causal responsibility does entail some kind of moral responsibility. Having conceded that much to the conservatives, I want to disentangle two aspects of moral responsibility which are confused in conservative arguments.

The first aspect, which I call *decision responsibility*, emerges as a strong theme in Carol Gilligan's interviews with women making the abortion decision.[11] Gilligan's women reveal that acceptance of causal responsibility means assuming a moral responsibility to make a decision or a series of decisions about your future relationship with the being whose existence you have directly brought about. The decision process is focused on questions such as whether you are in a position adequately to care for it, both now when it is in the fetal stage and, more importantly, when it is an independent being; how and whether it can be integrated into your life and the lives of others, for example other children, whose lives will also be significantly affected by your decision; whether you feel yourself able or prepared to provide the physical and emotional care and nurturance needed in order for both fetus and child to flourish. What emerges from these discussions is that the assumption of moral responsibility in pregnancy cannot be construed just in terms of responsibility toward the fetus but has a wider focus on the self, on relations with significant others, and on a person's other commitments and projects. When responsibility is construed in such a way, it is clear that exercising moral responsibility in no way entails a commitment to maternity and that the choice of abortion is in many cases the morally responsible decision.

The second aspect of moral responsibility in pregnancy, which I call *parental responsibility,* is the one which a person assumes when a commitment has been made to maternity.[12] This kind of assumption involves a responsibility not just to maintaining the existence of the fetus, nor even just a commitment to providing the care and nurturance needed for it to flourish, but a commitment to bringing into existence a future child. Often, though not necessarily, it also involves a commitment to long-term care and nurturance of that future child. My claim is that the decision to abort is a decision, for whatever reason, that one is not prepared to bring such a child into existence.

It should be pointed out here that, with respect to all aspects of responsibility, the situation of men and women in pregnancy at least is asymmetrical. The asymmetry is that while men and women are equally responsible for pregnancy in the causal sense, causal responsibility and decision responsibility are in effect completely separable for men, but inseparable for women. This is because a woman's bodily connection with the fetus makes causal responsibility and hence decision responsibility inescapable for her.[13] On the other hand, men's bodily alienation from the consequences of their actions and from the physical, psychic, and emotional experience of pregnancy means that they may be in a position where they are either unaware of their causal responsibility for the existence of the fetus or *choose* not to acknowledge their causal responsibility or assume decision responsibility.

A sensitivity to this difference illuminates two important points. First, if causal and decision responsibility are inseparable for women, then pregnancy cannot be thought of simply as a merely natural event which just *happens* to women and in relation to which they are passive. Although pregnancy certainly involves biological processes that are beyond the woman's control, these processes are always mediated by the cultural meanings of pregnancy, by the woman's personal and social context, and by the way she constitutes herself in response to these factors through the decisions she makes. In other words, pregnancy is never simply a biological process; it is always an active process of shaping for oneself a bodily and a moral perspective.[14] For this reason, the moral issues associated with pregnancy and abortion cannot be viewed in abstraction from the first-person perspective of the woman concerned.

Second, because of the particularity of the woman's situation in pregnancy, in cases of conflict over abortion ultimately it should be up to the woman to decide whether or not she will choose abortion.[15] To say this does not imply, however, that in situations where men are aware of and do acknowledge causal responsibility, they should have no say in an abortion decision. In such circumstances, because the decision made will obviously affect their autonomy, they should also be party to and involved in decision responsibility and, where appropriate, parental responsibility. Indeed, after birth they may assume most, or even all, parental responsibility. Nevertheless, prior to birth the impact on their autonomy of any decision is very different from its impact on the autonomy of the woman. This is why in cases of conflict the woman's decision should prevail.

Two objections are likely to be raised at this point. First, it is argued that a woman may also choose to relinquish moral responsibility, for example to others through adoption, and abortion *is* just a relinquishing of moral responsibility for the fetus'. From the preceding discussion, it should be clear that this objection conflates the two senses of moral responsibility distinguished here. Deciding against assuming parental responsibility does not mean that one has relinquished moral responsibility, not even for the fetus. For no matter what a woman decides—maternity, abortion, or adoption—she is still responsible to herself, to others, and to the child if there is one for the decision she has made. Further, as I have already pointed out, the decision to abort is often the most morally responsible course of action.

The second objection is that I have placed a great deal of moral weight on a decision process which in some cases just never occurs, for some women's lives are so chaotic and so little under their control that they cannot be said to be making any autonomous decisions about their own welfare, let alone about the welfare of any fetus that may be developing inside their body. My response to this objection, as I have already indicated, is to say that I would not attribute moral responsibility to a woman in such a situation. However, given the difficulty of actually deciding, in any given case, whether or not a woman does have any moral responsibility for a pregnancy, what the objection forces us to recognize is that a distinction needs to be made between our moral assessment of a situation and the matter of legal sanctions. Although I have argued that the decision to continue with a pregnancy entails some kind of parental responsibility, this is quite different from claiming that a woman should be legally liable for the fetus[1] welfare. Arguments to this effect must be vigorously resisted for they wrongly presume that fetuses are the moral and legal equivalents of women. In fact, as Warren has argued, "There is room for only one person with full and equal [legal] rights inside a single human skin".[16]

While this analysis of responsibility still leaves unanswered questions about the intrinsic moral status of the fetus, it does tend to suggest that, at least in part, its moral status depends on the relational properties it has with others and that the abortion issue cannot adequately be broached if we focus on intrinsic properties alone.[17] This relational aspect of the fetus' moral standing is best captured through the notion of moral guardianship. I want to suggest that although a fetus cannot be a bearer of full moral rights because, as I shall argue in the next section, it lacks the requisite intrinsic properties (namely person-hood), nevertheless in a context in which some one or more members of the moral community have decided to take parental responsibility for its future well-being, it has moral significance by virtue of its relations with her or them. We might say that in such a case it has de facto significance through her or them, until such a point when it can be considered a full moral being in its own right. This significance does not guarantee the fetus a "right to life" that over-rides all other possible competing claims, but rather provides some grounds for the fetus' claims to nurturance and care, that is, guardianship, from the woman who bears it and protection from harm from others.

In this context it should be noted that, once again, the situation of men and women with regard to moral guardianship is inescapably asymmetrical in preg-nancy. A man, no matter how well-intentioned, cannot act as the primary guardian of an in utero fetus. The reason for this asymmetry is not hard to discern—namely, the physical inseparability of the fetus from the woman—but its moral implications are often overlooked. The main implications are that, as I argued earlier, in cases of conflict it should be the woman who has the right to decide the fate of the fetus; moreover, this asymmetry makes it clear that, as Warren has argued, the event of birth is morally significant.[18] Its significance lies in the fact that at birth the infant becomes a member of the human moral community in its own right because its relationship with its mother and other human beings changes significantly. Not only is its body now separate from that of its mother, but it no longer needs to stand in a relation of moral and physical dependence on her in particular. Any responsible human adult will now be able to provide it with the care, nurturance, and moral protection required for it to flourish.

Having assessed the relational moral status of the fetus, I want now to justify my earlier claim that causal responsibility for the existence of the fetus entails decision responsibility because the fetus is a morally significant being. A useful starting point for this discussion is Warren's account of fetal status.

Fetal status and potentiality

If, following Warren, we distinguish between "human beings" and "persons" and argue that only persons can be members of the moral community, then it seems clear that the fetus is not a bearer of moral rights in the same sense that a person is and so does not have the same "right to life" as a person.[19] Nevertheless, as Warren herself argues with respect to infants, it does not follow from the fact that because anyone who is a person is entitled to strong moral protections, it is wrong to extend moral protections to beings that are not persons.[20] The more personlike the being, the more it should be treated as a person. The question arises therefore of how far advanced since conception a human being needs to be before it begins to have a right to life by virtue of being *like* a person—that is, at what stage should we start treating a fetus *as if* it were a person? On this point Warren in her earlier paper claims that the fetus of seven or eight months is no more personlike, or even less personlike, than the average fish and thus should not be treated as a person. For although, like the fish, the late-term fetus is sentient, sentience is not sufficient for personhood. Contra Thomson, she thus concludes that "whether or not it would be *indecent* (whatever that means) for a woman in her seventh month to obtain an abortion just to avoid having to postpone a trip to Europe, it would not, in itself, be *immoral*, and therefore it ought to be permitted."[21]

Warren's comparison between fetuses and fish occurs in the context of a discussion of the nature of personhood. The intention of the comparison is to show that while the fetus is indeed a member of the human species, as far as personhood and hence claims to rights are concerned, the fetus is morally on a par with a fish. With respect to driving home the distinction between human beings and persons, I do not dispute the effectiveness of Warren's comparison. However, I want to suggest that the metaphor is problematic for two reasons. First, it invites us to ignore the fact that, contingent though it may be, personhood is constituted by a complex of properties that supervene on a specific physical constitution.[22] Yet despite its contingency, or perhaps because of it, I believe that this fact is morally significant. Second, although the fetus/fish metaphor should not be read as providing a model of the relationship between a woman and a fetus, it has the serious, if unintended, effect of downplaying the moral significance and particularly of this relationship. In particular, it has the effect of deemphasizing both the woman's role as moral guardian and her parental responsibility for the present and future well-being of the fetus. The force of the feminist defense of abortion must lie in its highlighting of the moral particularity of the relationship between a woman and a fetus.

On the question of fetal status and potentiality, my claim is that fetuses are morally significant beings by virtue of the fact that they are potential persons. This makes them morally different in kind from fish. However, I think it is plausible to suggest that the moral value of the fetus[1] potential personhood is not static, but changes during the course of a normal pregnancy. This is because potential for personhood is not the only thing that bestows moral status on the being with that potentiality. Rather, the moral value of a being's potential personhood is related to the physical or biological basis of the potentiality; in particular, it is grounded in the degree of complexity and development of this physical basis. Thus the more physically complex and developed the being is, the more value we attribute to its potential for personhood. There are two ways in which this claim could be developed. One way would accept an on/off view of potentiality and argue that potential for personhood remains constant although its moral significance changes. On this view conceptus and late-term fetus both have the same potentiality, but the moral value of those beings is different because the physical basis of the potentiality is different. In the one case we have a clump of undifferentiated cells; in the other a highly complex organism. Thus, in the one case we have a being very far from being able to actualize its potentialities because it lacks the very physical basis to do so; in the other we have a being fairly close to being able to actualize its potentialities to the extent that the physical basis of those potentialities is highly developed.[23] Another way would be to question the on/off view of potentiality and to argue that potential for personhood itself changes as the fetus develops physically.[24]

For my purposes here nothing hinges on the differences between these positions. But what is appealing about the general suggestion is that it enables us to agree with Warren's criteria of personhood while nevertheless resisting the counterintuitive implications of these criteria—namely, that a being has no intrinsic moral significance unless it is a person and that there is no important moral difference between a conceptus and a late-term fetus. For now it can be argued that the intrinsic moral status of the fetus changes in direct relation to its changing physical basis. Thus, at least in terms of its intrinsic properties, an early stage fetus does not have great value. With respect to a highly developed fetus, although it is not a being with full moral rights, its gradually increasing moral significance warrants our treating it, in most circumstances at least, *as if* it were such a being.

Combining this view with the guardianship view outlined earlier, we get the idea that the moral position of the fetus changes over the course of pregnancy. At the early stages its moral standing is defined in relational terms, because it is a being with moral significance for the woman in whose body it develops and who acts as its moral guardian. As the fetus develops physically, however, its

intrinsic moral significance increases. Its moral standing is less and less dependent on its relational properties with the woman in whose body it develops and
more and more tied to its own intrinsic value. This does not mean, however,
that the fetus is *ever* the moral equivalent of the woman. Hence in cases where
the fetus' continued existence severely threatens the woman's physical or mental survival, her interests should always prevail up until the moment of birth. It
does suggest, however, that late-term abortion is morally different from early
abortion and that they cannot be justified on the same grounds.

On the question of guardianship, I suggested here that the rationale behind
Warren's defense of abortion (namely that the fetus is not a person), particularly in the context of the fetus/fish comparison, has the effect of downplaying the moral significance of the woman's parental responsibility for the present
and future well-being of the fetus. This effect is reinforced by Warren's claim,
which she justifies on the grounds of a woman's right to bodily autonomy, that
a decision to abort is morally permissible up until the moment of birth. For
now it looks as though the fetus is a potential threat to the woman's bodily
autonomy up until the moment of birth, rather than a being in relation to
whom the woman has a unique bodily and moral connection. In the next
section I shall argue that this view is based on a flawed conception of bodily
autonomy. Here I simply want to point out that in pregnancy the assumption of
parental responsibility necessarily involves a certain commitment of one's body.
In other words, the decision to continue a pregnancy (and presumably by seven
months some prior decision has been made) is a decision to assume responsibility (even if only for nine months) for the well-being of the fetus, and this
entails providing bodily nurturance for it, perhaps even at some bodily risk to
yourself. Now obviously there are limits to this risk. I am not suggesting that
women have responsibility to the fetus whatever the risk. As I have already
indicated, I am also not suggesting that parties other than the woman, for
example the medical establishment or the state-legal apparatus, have a right to
determine the limits of that risk. Like many other feminists, including Warren, I
am alarmed by the recent movements advocating both so-called "fetal rights"
and the introduction of charges of "fetal abuse" against women who do not do
what is required to nurture the fetus in the uterus. Further, the whole question
of what is "required" for adequate nurturance is open to much interpretation
against women's autonomy as persons. Nevertheless, I think that my accounts
of potentiality, guardianship, and responsibility explain why there is a genuine
moral requirement upon a woman to protect and nurture a fetus once she has

assumed parental responsibility for its future well-being, without that requirement involving any infringement of her autonomy. In this context it should be
noted that Warren's downplaying of the question of responsibility also fails to
stress men's obligations with respect to a pregnancy.

Pregnant embodiment and bodily autonomy

I have argued so far that, at least in the early stages of its development, the moral
standing of a fetus is dependent upon its relationship with the woman who
bears it and who acts as its moral guardian. In terms of its own intrinsic
properties, its moral standing is not particularly significant. This is a necessary
condition for the permissibility of abortion, but it is not sufficient for it fails to
explain why the availability of abortion is necessary for the moral autonomy of
women and hence why a restriction on its accessibility violates their autonomy.
In this section I attempt to explain and justify this claim. From my discussion it
will also become clear why, in order to secure women's autonomy, abortion
must be understood as fetal death rather than fetal evacuation.

What has emerged so far is that in order to understand the kind of autonomy
that is exercised by women in pregnancy and abortion we must be attentive to
the moral particularity of pregnancy. As we have seen, a number of different
factors make pregnancy morally unique. To begin, pregnancy is not simply a
biological event with respect to which women are passive; rather, it is an active
process and a social process that places women in a situation of moral responsibility, which I earlier called decision responsibility. This responsibility is due
in part to the fetus' potential moral significance, but it is also due to the fact that
the decision to commit or not to commit oneself to the existence of such a
future person has far-reaching implications for the woman's own life as well as,
possibly, for the lives of others—for example, the "father" of the possible future
child; other children, relatives, friends; and so on. But pregnancy is also morally
unique because the physical connection between the woman and the fetus, and
the physical processes that occur during pregnancy, give rise to a unique bodily
perspective.

In what follows I shall draw on a phenomenological account of pregnant
embodiment in order to give an account of the kind of reflective bodily perspective that emerges from the experience of pregnancy. I shall also suggest that
the experience of moral responsibility in pregnancy, which I have already detailed, is mediated by this reflective bodily perspective, which both structures
and points to the moral particularity of the relationship between woman and

fetus, especially to the fact that this relationship and the responsibilities it entails cannot be conceived of as extrinsic to the woman's subjectivity. I want to make it clear that this phenomenological description is not a description of the subjective feelings of individual women, but is rather a normative and reflective apprehension of the way in which conscious experience is structured by our (bodily) situations, perspectives, and modes of perception. The phenomenological experience I describe is therefore not meant to be an empirical description of the way in which all women experience or feel about their pregnancies, since women's individual bodily perspectives, feelings, and experiences depend on a wide range of factors, including the cultural, social, and historical context in which they live their lives.[25]

My suggestion is that although in some ways (for example, biologically) it makes sense to speak of the fetus as a separate being from the woman, in other ways (for example in terms of talking of a conflict of rights), it makes no sense at all especially in the early stages of pregnancy.[26] Phenomenologically, the experience of pregnancy, particularly in the early stages, is unique in the sense that it defies a sharp opposition between self and other, between the inside and the outside of the body. From the perspective of the woman, there *is* no clear-cut boundary between herself and the fetus, between her body boundaries and the body boundaries of the fetus. The fetus, to the extent that it is experienced as part of the woman's body, is also experienced as part of her self, but as a part that is also other than herself. On the one hand, it is another being, but it is another being growing inside her body, a being whose separateness is not fully realized as such by her. This is the case even with an unwanted pregnancy. The uniqueness and intimacy of this kind of relationship, one where the distinction between self and other is blurred, suggests that the welfare of the fetus, at least early on, is not easily separable from that of the woman. The fetus is not simply an entity extrinsic to her which happens to be developing inside her body and which she desires either to remove or to allow to develop. It is a being, both inseparable and yet separate from her, both part of and yet soon to be independent from her, whose existence calls into question her own present and future identity.

The changing phenomenology of pregnancy also concurs with the account I have given of fetal status, for it seems to me that one of the main reasons for the experience I have described is that in early pregnancy, although the woman's body is undergoing massive changes, the fetus itself is not very physically developed. The fetus' separateness is thus neither physically well established nor is it felt as such by the woman. As pregnancy continues, as the fetus develops physically, a triple process occurs. First, from the perspective of the woman, the fetus becomes more and more physically differentiated from her and her own body boundaries alter. Second, this gradual physical differentiation (which becomes very pronounced as soon as the fetus starts moving around—perhaps explaining why "quickening" used to be considered morally significant) is paralleled by and gives rise to a gradual psychic differentiation, in the experience of the woman, between herself and the fetus. In other words, as the fetus' body develops, it seems to become less and less a part of the woman and of her body although, as psychoanalysis reminds us, the psychic experiences of unity and differentiation continue to resonate for both mother and child right through infancy and early childhood. Third, physical and psychic differentiation are usually accompanied by an increasing emotional attachment of the woman to the fetus, an attachment that is based both in her physical connection with the fetus and in an anticipation of her future relationship with a separate being who is also intimately related to her.

From the reflective perspective of the woman, the fetus thus has a double and ambivalent status. On the one hand, it is experienced as interior to her own subjectivity, and this sense of interiority is grounded in the bodily connection between the woman and the fetus. On the other hand, this experience of interiority and connection is interrupted by an awareness that, if the pregnancy continues, this being which is now a part of her will become a separate being for whose welfare she is morally responsible. But this awareness itself arises in part from the woman's bodily experiences, for example, from the changes to her body shape and from feelings of the strangeness of her body to her which remind her of the other being growing within her. I think it is this double character of the fetus' bodily and moral relationship to the woman that explains why questions of responsibility are central to the experience of pregnancy and why the right of determination over the fate of the fetus is essential for a woman's autonomy.[27]

I think this reflective perspective also explains why it is a mistake to construe bodily autonomy in pregnancy and abortion simply as a matter of preserving the integrity of one's body boundaries. It is this kind of understanding of bodily autonomy that seems to inform the views of Thomson and Warren, at least in her early paper, who construe the right to bodily integrity along the lines of a property-right. The idea seems to be that a woman has a right to preserve the integrity of her body boundaries and to control what happens in and to her body in the same way as she has a right to dispose of her property as she sees fit, and that the denial to women of access to abortion might be said to be akin to a system of coverture. I think this idea is quite explicit in such feminist slogans as "Keep *your* filthy laws off *my* body" and in some of Thomson's metaphors, for example, the metaphor of the body as a house. Now it seems to me that underlying this view of the body is the mistaken idea that I am the owner of my body and my body parts and that, as their owner, I can dispose of them, use them, or contract them out for use as I see fit. This view of the body often underlies defenses of surrogacy, but I think it is also evident in Thomson's assumptions about pregnancy. In her argument pregnancy emerges as a kind of contract between the woman and the fetus such that she contracts with it for it to use her body for the required period until it is able to survive without her. Thus in Thomson's violinist example the idea seems to be that the unwanted fetus is attempting to use a woman's body without her having contracted with it to do so, and it is this which makes abortion permissible. A similar kind of presumption seems to be operating in Warren's view that the fetus represents a potential threat to the woman's bodily autonomy up to the moment of birth.

For the remainder of this article I shall argue that this conception of bodily autonomy, and the rights-based model which provides the framework for it, are seriously flawed. My first set of objections to this way of defending abortion is that it misrepresents both the nature of pregnancy and the woman-fetus relationship. As a result, it is unable to come to terms with the question of moral responsibility in pregnancy. The second and connected objection is that it justifies the demand for abortion in terms of a right to an evacuated uterus, rather than a right to autonomy with respect to one's own life. This misrepresents the nature of the abortion decision. These two objections are explained in the next two subsections.

Bodily autonomy, subjectivity, and responsibility

It seems that underlying the property-contract model of bodily autonomy is a very inert view of pregnancy in which pregnancy is represented as a purely biological process with respect to which women are passive. It is as though, having agreed to the terms of the contract, the woman then simply allows her body to be used by the fetus. But this view of pregnancy blinds us to the fact that the relationship between the woman and the fetus is a special relationship of a very particular nature. The fetus is not a stranger contracting with the woman for use of her body but another, not yet separate, being growing within her body, a being implicated in her own sense of self and whose very existence places her in a situation of moral responsibility.

However, if we take seriously both the issue of responsibility in pregnancy and the kind of reflective bodily perspective that I have argued emerges from the process of pregnancy, then pregnancy seems to defy making any sharp distinction between a passive, unconscious, biological process and an active, conscious, rational process. To a large extent, the biological processes occurring in a woman's body are beyond her control; nevertheless, as I have already argued, these processes are always mediated by the cultural meanings of pregnancy, by the woman's personal and social context, and by the way she constitutes herself in response to these factors through the decisions she makes. Thus coming to terms with pregnancy and its implications, taking responsibility of whatever kind for the future of the fetus, are the activities of an autonomous moral agent. Bodily autonomy in pregnancy and abortion thus cannot be construed simply as the right to bodily integrity. Rather, it is a question of being able to shape for oneself an integrated bodily perspective, a perspective by means of which a woman can respond to the bodily processes she experiences in a way with which she identifies, and which is consistent with the decision she makes concerning her future moral relationship with the fetus.

To think that the question of autonomy in abortion is just a question about preserving the integrity of one's body boundaries, and to see the fetus merely as an occupant of the woman's uterus, is thus to divorce women's bodies from their subjectivities. Ironically, it comes close to regarding women's bodies simply as fetal containers—the very charge that many feminists have leveled against the fetal rights movement. If, however, we see our subjectivities as constituted through the constitution of our bodily perspectives so that, following Merleau-Ponty, we see the body as our point of view upon the world, then my body is no more my property than I myself am my own property.[28] Rather, my body is my mode of being-in-the-world. Consequently, changes to my body or to my perceptions of my body image must affect my relation to the world. The experience of pregnant embodiment—that is, the gradual differentiation and development from within her own body of another being which is now a part of herself—thus affects a woman's mode of being-in-the-world both physically and morally and, as a consequence, her sense of self. She is now no longer just herself but herself and another, but this other is not yet separate from herself. It is because of this psychic and bodily connectedness between the woman and the fetus that in pregnancy questions about the fate of the fetus cannot be separated from the issue of a woman's right to self-determination.

Evacuation and abortion

If, as I have argued, the early-stage fetus is morally insignificant (in terms of its own intrinsic properties) and its identity and very existence are as yet indistinguishable from that of the woman, it becomes nonsensical to speak of a conflict of rights between them because we cannot talk about the needs and rights of the fetus in abstraction from those of the woman.[29] The idea of such a conflict only makes any sense later in pregnancy where the fetus is physically well developed and differentiated from the woman and where this physical basis now grounds a definite and significant moral value. Combining my earlier discussion of the moral insignificance of the early-stage fetus with my claim that the early-stage fetus is phenomenologically and psychically experienced by the woman as both part and not part of herself, thus grounds the moral permissibility of securing its death. At present, the fetus is in itself a morally insignificant part of herself, but it is a part of herself which, if the pregnancy continues, will become a separate, independent, and significant being for whose future existence she will be required to take parental responsibility and to whom she will become increasingly emotionally attached. What the abortion decision involves is a decision that this part of herself should not *become* a being in relation to whom such questions of parental responsibility and emotional attachment arise. In other words, abortion is not a matter of wanting to kill *this particular being*, which is, after all, as yet indistinguishable from oneself. It is rather a matter of not wanting there to *be* a future child, so intimately related to oneself, for which one either has to take responsibility or give up to another.

Because property-contract models of bodily autonomy are inattentive to the phenomenological experience of pregnancy and ignore questions of moral responsibility they misrepresent the nature of this decision. If the demand for abortion is just the demand to control one's own body and use its parts as one sees fit, then abortion cannot involve the right to choose whether or not to bring a child into existence but only the right to evacuate a fetus from one's body. While Thomson and Warren explicitly acknowledge this as an implication of their account of bodily autonomy, they do not defend the position to which they are committed. In her discussion of abortion in *Ethics and Human Reproduction* Christine Overall does, however, attempt to defend this position even though she is explicitly critical of a property-contract view of women's bodies. My argument is that such a position is inconsistent with a concern for women's autonomy.[30] In what follows I shall develop this argument via a critical analysis of Overall's discussion.

Overall argues that abortion consists of two conceptually and morally distinct events which, though inseparable in current gynecological practice may yet, with the advancing state of technology, become separable: (1) evacuation of the fetus from the uterus and (2) destruction of the fetus. Overall's argument is that while (1) is morally permissible, (2) is not. In other words, if the fetus could be kept alive in some kind of incubator or if some form of fetal transplant and adoption were possible—that is, the evacuation of the fetus from one's woman's uterus and its implantation in the uterus of another—then such procedures would be morally required.

Overall's argument, which is very similar to a double-effect argument, involves a reconstrual of the alleged rights conflict in abortion. Where the original formulation is a conflict between (a) the fetus' right to life, and (b) a woman's right to bodily autonomy, she reconstrues this, in terms of an absence of rights, as a conflict between (c) the pregnant woman (or anyone else, e.g., a physician) who has no right to kill the embryo/fetus, and (d) the embryo/fetus which has no right to occupancy of its mother's (or anyone else's) uterus. Overall's claim is that the right to bodily autonomy reconstrued as (d) does not entail (2). (d) involves a simple taking-over of Thomson's formulation without further argumentation. Overall's main argument in defense of (c) is an appeal to the fetus' potential personhood, but "appeal" is all it is because Overall does not discuss the criteria for personhood nor explain how we should understand the claim that fetuses are potential persons. In addition, she simply assumes that fetuses at all stages of development have the same moral significance.[31]

Overall is aware that her position gives rise to many difficult questions: Ought we to save all aborted fetuses? Should we try to adopt them out were that possible? What if fetal adoption caused more suffering for women or for fetuses? She attempts to avoid some of these and to resolve the conflict between conflicting rights (c) and (d) by arguing that they apply to different periods of pregnancy. Hence right (d) may be regarded as overriding in early pregnancy (with abortion then resulting in the foreseeable but unintended death of the fetus), whereas right (c) may be regarded as overriding in late pregnancy.

While I agree with Overall that, in most cases, it is morally indefensible to demand the death of a late-term fetus, the problem with her argument is that she offers no reasons why this should be the case, nor does she offer an explanation why, if, as she thinks, there is no significant difference in moral standing between a conceptus and a late-term fetus, the foreseeable consequence of the fetus' death should be any more allowable early in pregnancy than later on. As I have shown, however, there are a number of reasons why there is a morally significant difference between a conceptus and a late-term fetus, and it is this difference that makes fetal death in early abortions morally permissible. I conclude then that Overall's defense of abortion as fetal evacuation fails.

More importantly, however, Overall's failure to make any significant moral discriminations between different stages of fetal development renders her "solution" to the conflict between (c) and (d) arbitrary and far too contingent upon what is technologically feasible. Were it to become possible to evacuate an early-stage fetus from the uterus of one woman and implant it into the uterus of another or to rear it in an incubator, Overall would be committed to the moral desirability of this procedure. Not only that, she would be committed to arguing that such a procedure, rather than abortion, is morally required. For the reasons outlined in this article, it seems to me disturbing that this outcome should seem to follow from a feminist defense of abortion. Apart from oversimplifying the complex issue of fetal status, this position ignores the fact that much more is at stake in the demand for abortion than the misconceived demand to dispose of or use one's own body parts as one sees fit. What is at issue is women's moral autonomy, an autonomy which, because of the specificity of women's embodiment, must include autonomy with respect to the fate of any fetus developing within her body. Because of the connection between the fetus, which is both part and not part of herself, and the woman's moral and bodily subjecthood, to allow the fate of the fetus to be settled by what is or is not technologically feasible once again removes from women what the availability of abortion helps make possible—the right to autonomous moral agency with respect to one's own life.

Conclusion: metaphors, experience and moral thinking

I shall conclude this discussion with some brief reflections on the methodological implications of the analysis I have given. A survey of the philosophical literature on abortion, including some of the feminist philosophical literature, shows that philosophical thinking on this topic has been dominated by bizarre metaphors and fantastic examples (Warren's fish, Tooley's kittens, Thomson's violinists, people-seeds, houses, and so on) and has given rise to abstruse metaphysical speculations about the nature of personal identity (Parfit). These examples and speculations have undoubtedly served to question certain common unreflective prejudices and to highlight the philosophical ramifications and complexities of some of the questions raised by abortion. Unfortunately, they have also contributed to the representation of pregnancy as a mere *event* that simply takes over women's lives and with respect to which women are passive. In addition, they have focused philosophical and moral reflection away from the contexts in which deliberations about abortion are usually made and away from the concerns and experiences that motivate those involved in the processes of deliberation. The result is that philosophical analyses of abortion often seem beside the point, if not completely irrelevant, to the lives of the countless women who daily not only have to make moral decisions about abortion but, more importantly, often face serious risks to their lives in contexts where abortion is not a safe and readily accessible procedure. While I do not pretend to have addressed the social, religious, political, and legal obstacles that give rise to this abhorrent situation, I do hope to have explained why the morality of abortion is not simply or even primarily about questions concerning personhood and fetal status but more fundamentally is about women's self-determination.

Notes

This article was first published in the *Australasian Journal of Philosophy* 70 (1992): 136–155, and is reprinted with permission. I am grateful to the editor of the journal and to anonymous referees for their comments on earlier versions of this article. Earlier versions were also read to the philosophy department at Monash University, the Philosophy Society at Princeton University, and a seminar on Legal and Conceptual Aspects of Abortion at the University of New South Wales. I would like to thank participants in those discussions for their comments. I would also like to thank the following people for their helpful discussions and/or comments: John Bigelow, John Burgess, Genevieve Lloyd, Michaelis Michael, Robert Pargetter, Peter Singer, Michael Smith, and C. L. Ten.

1   My argument in this part of the article refers to Mary Anne Warren's paper "On the Moral and Legal Status of Abortion," in R. Wasserstrom, ed., *Today's Moral Problems* (London: Macmillan, 1975). In a very recent paper, to which I refer in more detail later, Warren's characterization of the fetus is markedly different although her basic position on a woman's right to bodily autonomy remains unaltered. See "The Moral Significance of Birth," *Hypatia* 4 (1989): 46–65. This paper is a modified version of an earlier paper with the same title that appeared in *Bioethics News*, Publication of the Centre for Human Bioethics, Monash University, vol. 7, no. 2, January 1988.

2   Judith Jarvis Thomson, "A Defense of Abortion," *Philosophy and Public Affairs*, 1 (1971): 47–66; Christine Overall, *Ethics and Human Reproduction* (Boston: Allen and Unwin, 1987), chs. 3, 4.

3   Steven Ross, "Abortion and the Death of the Fetus," *Philosophy and Public Affairs* 11 (1982): 232–245.

4   I discuss the question of men's responsibility below. Given this account of causal respon-
    sibility, a woman is, of course, not causally responsible in the case of rape. In cases where a
    woman cannot and cannot reasonably be expected to foresee the consequences of her actions
    (e.g., if she is a minor or mentally disabled) or if her actions were performed under duress (the
    distinction between rape and consent is not as hard and fast as many would think), or if she
    cannot be said to be acting autonomously (e.g., in a case of drug addiction or alcoholism or
    some other dependency), I would argue that, although a woman may have some causal
    responsibility for the outcome of her actions, she cannot be considered to be morally respon-
    sible for this outcome.

5   Somewhat surprisingly, some feminists have argued for a similar view. See Hilde and James
    Lindemann Nelson, "Cutting Motherhood in Two: Some Suspicions Concerning Surrogacy,"
    Hypatia 4 (1989): 85–94.

6   Warren, "On the Moral and Legal Status of Abortion"; Michael Tooley, "Abortion and Infan-
    ticide," *Philosophy and Public Affairs* 2 (1972): 37–65.

7   The violinist example seeks to show that a person has no moral obligation to sustain the life of
    a famous violinist who has been attached to her without her consent, and whose survival is
    dependent on being connected to her circulatory system for nine months. The Henry Fonda
    example involves the case of a person who is dying but would be revived by the touch of Henry
    Fonda's hand on her brow. The example seeks to show that a person does not necessarily have
    a right to whatever is required to ensure her survival. See Thomson, "A Defence of Abortion."
    I discuss the problem with such examples in the final section of this article.

8   Warren, "On the Moral and Legal Status of Abortion"; Joel Feinberg, "Abortion," in Tom
    Regan, ed., *Matters of Life and Death* (New York: Random House, 1980).

9   In this example people-seeds are seeds that blow in through house windows like dust, take
    root in carpets, and then grow into people who demand food and shelter!

10 I have in mind here Thomson's discussion of the woman who at seven months requests an
    abortion in order to avoid having to postpone an overseas trip. Thomson realizes that her
    argument does not allow her to claim that such a request would be immoral, so she resorts to
    the claim that it would be indecent. This issue aside, Thomson's example is somewhat offen-
    sive in its presentation of women's moral attitude toward abortion. Women who seek abor-
    tions at this stage of pregnancy are usually those whose health is in some way gravely threat-
    ened by continuation of the pregnancy, or those who, due to drug addiction, mental disability,
    or some other such reason, cannot be said ever to have made a moral decision with regard to
    their pregnancies.

11 Carol Gilligan, *In a Different Voice* (Cambridge, Mass.: Harvard University Press, 1982). It
    should be noted here that the kinds of moral reflection in which these women engage is in part
    made possible by the fact that they do have reproductive choice.

12 As I have indicated, decision responsibility is a process, not a single decision. Thus a woman
    may change her mind a number of times before finally assuming parental responsibility. She
    may also change her mind after having assumed it. For reasons that I explain below, I think
    there is a significant *moral* difference between such a change of mind in the first trimester or
    early in the second trimester and a change of mind during the latter half of pregnancy, except
    of course where such a change is made for medical reasons or because of fetal deformity

discoverable only by amniocentesis during the second trimester. It does not follow from this, however, that women should be *legally* prevented from obtaining abortions for other reasons later in pregnancy. I discuss the distinction between moral and legal responsibility later in this chapter.

13   I discuss the nature of this bodily connection in detail in the last section of this chapter.

14   I develop this point in more detail in the last section.

15   I have in mind here recent cases in the United Kingdom and Australia where men have attempted to obtain court orders, on the grounds of paternal right, to prevent women from obtaining abortion. My analysis of the asymmetry in the positions of men and women with respect to responsibility in pregnancy should make it clear why feminists have been so outraged by the men's presumption in these cases that they should be able to overrule the decisions of the women concerned.

16   My insert. Warren, "Moral Significance of Birth," p. 63.

17   Warren also criticizes what she calls "the intrinsic-properties assumption" on the grounds that it cannot account for the moral significance of birth. Ibid., pp. 47–56.

18   Ibid., p. 56.

19   Warren, "On the Moral and Legal Status of Abortion." Warren supports this distinction by outlining five criteria for personhood, specifying that a person need not satisfy all these criteria but that a being which satisfied none of them could not be considered a person. The five criteria are: (1) consciousness (of objects and events external and/or internal to the being), in particular the capacity to feel pain; (2) reasoning (the *developed* capacity to solve new and relatively complex problems); (3) self-motivated activity (activity that is relatively independent of either genetic or direct external control); (4) the capacity to communicate, by whatever means, messages of an indefinite variety of types, that is, not just with an indefinite number of possible contents, but on indefinitely many possible topics; and (5) the presence of self-concepts and self-awareness, either individual or racial, or both.

20   Warren, "Moral Significance of Birth." I follow Warren here in using the term *person* because I think that in the context of abortion the distinction between human beings and persons is important to maintain. However, I am not happy with the legalistic and individualist connotations of the term which tend to downplay the intersubjective processes of development by means of which infants become self-conscious subjects.

21   Warren, "On the Moral and Legal Status of Abortion," p. 133.

22   In stressing the connection between the development of subjectivity and physical development I am not denying the significance of the social relationships in the context of which these developments must occur.

23   This argument is a simplified version of an argument of John Bigelow and Robert Pargetter. See "Morality, Potential Persons and Abortion," *American Philosophical Quarterly* 25 (1988): 173–181.

24   An argument for this view is presented by Michaelis Michael in "The Moral Significance of Potential for Personhood" (unpublished paper, Monash University, 1986). His view is that the potential for personhood of a being can be expressed as a function, from situations the being is (normally) in, to the probabilities of its giving rise to a person from those situations. We have great potential when we have one function dominating another.

25   My account here builds on psychoanalytic insights into the mother-child relation, on some of the descriptions of pregnancy and maternity in the work of Julia Kristeva, on Iris Young's phenomenology of pregnant embodiment, and on my own a posteriori reconstructions. See Julia Kristeva, "Motherhood according to Giovanni Bellini," in *Desire in Language* (Oxford: Blackwell, 1980), and Kristeva, "Stabat Mater," in T. Moi, ed., *The Kristeva Reader* (Oxford: Blackwell, 1986); Iris Marion Young, "Pregnant Embodiment: Subjectivity and Alienation," *Journal of Medicine and Philosophy* 9 (1984): 45–62.

26   The rights-based model has also been criticized on different but related grounds by other feminists. See Janet Farrell Smith, "Rights-Conflict, Pregnancy and Abortion," in Carol Gould, ed., *Beyond Domination* (Totowa, N.J.: Rowman and Allanheld, 1984), pp. 265–273.

27   At this point I would like to respond to an objection that is often made against the view I have proposed here. It could be argued that the woman's experience of the fetus as part of herself and as interior to her subjectivity is simply mistaken. So why should any moral weight be given to this experience? How is it different, for example, from the experience of a slave owner who regards his/her slaves as a part of him/herself and thinks that because of this he/she has a right to determine their fate? My response to this suggestion is that these cases are completely disanalogous, and for two reasons. First, I have argued that a necessary condition for the permissibility of abortion is that the fetus, especially in the early stages of pregnancy, has little moral value in and of itself, although it may have a great deal of value for the woman in whose body it develops. This is not merely an arbitrary claim, like the claim of the slave owner who may think that his/her slaves have little moral value in and of themselves. Rather it is justified by the fact that the fetus simply does not yet have the capacities that ground the moral worth of persons, and by the fact that the fetus' possible potential for personhood has little significance until those capacities are close to being actualized.

But, second, this objection ignores what I have been insisting on throughout this article, namely that the relationship of the woman to the fetus is morally unique. It is not a relationship of domination and subordination and inhuman ownership, as in the case of the slave owner. Rather, it is a relationship in which one human being grows and develops *inside* the body of another, and in which the moral significance of the fetus is in part bound up with its significance for the woman. The moral particularity of this situation, in other words, is grounded in the nature of the bodily connection between woman and fetus. The woman's sense of the fetus as a part of herself is thus not arbitrary. It arises, as I have tried to show, from her own reflective bodily perspective and from the kind of moral reflection to which pregnancy gives rise.

Certainly it is possible to think up all kinds of examples in which the relationship between the woman and the fetus might have been different, as in Thomson's examples. But my point is that these examples cannot give us an adequate understanding of the moral complexities of the issues raised by pregnancy and abortion precisely because they overlook the context out of which these complexities arise, namely the bodily and moral connection between the woman and the fetus.

28   I am drawing here on Maurice Merleau-Ponty's discussion of the body in *The Phenomenology of Perception* (1945), translated by Colin Smith (London: Routledge and Kegan Paul, 1962).

29   This does not mean, of course, that we cannot talk of what is physically harmful or beneficial to the development of the fetus.

30 Anne Donchin has expressed similar worries about the implications of Overall's position. See her review essay "The Growing Feminist Debate over the New Reproductive Technologies," *Hypatia* 4 (1989): 136–149.

31 Overall offers three supposedly analogous cases which are supposed to back up this appeal and to show why the right to bodily autonomy, reconstrued as (d), does not entail a woman's right to demand (2), that is, the destruction of the fetus. The problem with these cases, however, is that Overall fails to make any moral discriminations between different stages of fetal development. The cases are as follows:

(A) If an aborted fetus lives, we have no right to kill it, although we are not morally obliged to keep it alive. Here Overall seems to be appealing to the acts and omissions doctrine, which in this context I would reject on compassionate grounds. If the fetus is likely to die and will presumably suffer more if simply allowed to die (which is pretty certain if we are talking about an abortion prior to twenty weeks), it seems morally preferable that we kill it.

(B) We have no right to kill premature babies in a case, for example, where the mother might have wanted an abortion but was prevented from obtaining one. But if there is no moral difference between a twenty-six-week premature baby and a twenty-six-week in utero fetus, it should be just as morally wrong to kill the fetus as the baby. Overall's argument here appeals to the claim that all fetuses, at whatever stage of development, are morally indistinguishable. I have already argued against this claim and have agreed that killing a late-term fetus is morally different from killing an early fetus, although I have also indicated that I would not rule it out a priori, for example, in cases where it is unlikely it would ever acquire the complex physical basis required for personhood. I would agree, though, with Overall that were it possible to abort a late-term fetus alive, in most cases where the fetus was likely to survive and become a healthy infant the mother would not have the right to kill it. Having said that, I would nevertheless take issue with Overall's claim that there is no moral difference between a twenty-six-week premature baby and a twenty-six-week in utero fetus, which assumes that birth has no moral significance.

(C) At the other end of the process, Overall claims that neither fetus nor embryo is the property of the parents. Thus, she argues, just as parents involved in in vitro fertilization programs should not have the right to demand the destruction of embryos, neither do women have the right to secure the death of the fetus. While I would agree with Overall that neither conceptus nor fetus is the property of its parents, I disagree that it is only on such grounds that we might regard it as their right to determine its fate. I don't want here to tackle the issue of the disposal of in vitro fertilization embryos and/or fetal tissue. Suffice it to say that Overall's argument once again trades on the unargued claim that fetuses at all stages of development have intrinsic moral worth as "potential" persons.

From bioethics to microethics: ethical debate and clinical medicine

Paul A. Komesaroff

Preface: bioethics versus clinical ethics

It is midnight in the emergency room of a country hospital. A patient is carried in by four attendants. He is angry and aggressive, shouting obscenities and struggling vigorously. It transpires that he is a prisoner in a local jail and that the attendants are warders. One of them claims that he has been behaving irrationally and needs medical attention; when approached, however, the patient becomes even more hostile and refuses to cooperate in any way.

Everyone will agree that this rather vivid and dramatic scenario raises issues of an ethical kind. What does not command assent, however, is just what these issues are. For example, when viewed from the standpoint of biomedical ethics or, as it is often called in the rapidly expanding literature in the field, *bioethics,* the problem appears rather differently than when viewed from that of clinical medicine. In the former case, the issues are relatively clear-cut, even if the solutions are not: they include the degree of autonomy the patient can exercise in these circumstances, balanced against the doctor's obligations of nonmalefi- cence and beneficence, and questions of justice, including the fairness and evenhandedness of the treatment of this particular individual. In the latter case, however, the key ethical question is not "How autonomous is this patient?" or "How can justice be maximized?" but simply "How are we going to deal with this clinical problem?" For the clinician, the task is to determine how to ap- proach the clinical predicament in all its complex and unpredictable detail: how to facilitate communication with a man who is likely to regard doctors and hospitals with suspicion and hostility, how to obtain the information necessary for a diagnosis, how to carry out decisions about investigative procedures and treatment, and so on. The job of the clinician, in other words, cannot be formulated in terms of broad principles, bioethical or otherwise, but only as a series of practical tasks. For him or her, this means that the major problem that must be addressed at the outset is how to engage this particular patient, with his distinctive history and special circumstances, in the peculiar and characteristic context of the clinic.

The emergency room again late at night. The patient is a middle-aged, non-English-speaking man, surrounded by his large, very concerned family. He complains, loudly and repeatedly of abdominal pain; however, he refuses to allow you to touch his abdomen in order to perform the appropriate physical examination, which he clearly regards as unnecessary.

Once again, the perspectives of the bioethicist and the clinician diverge. For the former, as previously, the case presents—at least in superficial terms—a relatively straightforward ethical problem. Is the patient legitimately exercising his autonomy in refusing to let you examine him? If he is, there is in all probability little else to be said. For the latter, however, while the problem is indeed an ethical one, it is of a somewhat different kind. Here, the issue concerns the form and texture of the communication between the doctor and the patient, having regard to both the cultural and personality factors at work. From the clinical viewpoint, the question is formulated not in terms of "autonomy" but, practically, in terms of the most appropriate way to approach the patient, to talk with him, to allay his fears, and to establish the common ground on which mutual decisions can be taken.

This chapter seeks to examine the differences between the approach to the ethical problems in medicine developed by contemporary bioethics and that inherent in the practice of clinical medicine.

Medical ethics today

In recent years there has been an explosion of interest in medical ethics. The dilemmas of modern medicine are now widely and vigorously discussed in the popular media, in the community at large, and in the medical literature. The curricula of almost all medical schools incorporate at least some teaching on the subject of the ethical issues associated with medical practice, and biomedical ethics has become a respectable field of study in its own right. There are at least six international journals devoted exclusively or predominantly to the field; there are graduate courses and dedicated research institutes devoted to defining and pursuing its problems. It is perhaps not too much of an exaggeration to say that bioethics now constitutes a substantial academic industry.

The enhanced interest in medical ethics represents a response to a perception in the community that medicine has somehow lost touch with its original purposes—that it has been transformed into an efficient instrument for achieving technical goals, with little regard to their human or social implications.[1] The development of rigorous methods of reflection on current practices, furthermore, has indeed gone some of the way to meeting that concern and, undeniably, has thereby produced some beneficial consequences. For example, at least partially as a result of these debates, doctors have become more aware of the conceptual issues implicit in decisions which they previously often made without deep consideration, and they have developed skills in critical reflection and argumentation. The medical profession in general has become more sensitive to community attitudes. At the same time, in the community generally, the complexity of medical practice has become more widely appreciated.

However, reflection on the ethical problems of medicine and biology has come to be largely dominated by a series of assumptions, conventions, and imperatives regarding the formulation of the questions to be considered and the methods of argument. This has given rise to some disquiet among many practicing clinicians, because the body of thought in question often appears to present the ethical discussions as abstract and divorced from the real concerns of doctors and patients, with many of the most important issues being obscured or passed over. Consequently, the ethical analysis does not always contribute to the actual decision-making process. Further, and possibly more importantly, both practicing clinicians and their patients often feel at a disadvantage—that they are in some way out of their depth—when talking about ethical issues, which are thus left to be dealt with in the technical domain of the philosophers.

There is a growing, if still incipient, recognition of the deficiencies of bioethics among both the medical and the philosophical communities. Indeed, there is now a substantial body of writing reflecting critically on bioethics and its philosophical foundations. This literature includes specific analyses from within bioethics itself,[2] critiques by practicing clinicians[3] or by philosophers working in the field of the ethics of medical practice but outside the paradigms of bioethics proper,[4] and reflections of a more global nature on the foundations of ethical theory.[5] Among the many criticisms that are advanced in these discussions are the claims that bioethics lacks a reliable theoretical foundation and that many of its arguments are circular. The question is also raised of the proper relationship between bioethics, which is concerned with complex issues covering many disciplines, and philosophical ethics, in its various forms, which has often been assumed—without sufficient justification, it is claimed—to provide a theoretical framework for the entire discourse.

It is not a concern of this essay to provide a detailed critique of bioethics, or even to offer an exhaustive list of the many standpoints from which it has been subjected to scrutiny. Instead, in what follows, some of its fundamental deficiencies will be outlined and some suggestions will be made regarding possible future directions for ethical reflections on medical practice.

My claim is that bioethics is deficient because it is unable to provide an adequate account of day-to-day decision making in medicine, as a result of which it cannot provide any substantial guidance for medical practice. I argue that this is not an accidental circumstance and cannot be blamed merely on the development of a "biomedical establishment" made up of philosophers, lawyers, theologians, and sociologists rather than of practicing clinicians.[6] Rather, the problem has its roots in the historical tradition from which contemporary philosophical ethics arose. It manifests itself not just in the conclusions of specific arguments but also, more fundamentally, in the ways in which the objects of the discipline are formulated and in the strategies of argumentation that are employed.

The subjects covered by the bioethical literature are already familiar and are of substantial public interest. This apparent familiarity is itself largely a product of the bioethical culture and indicates one of its most pernicious effects, which has been to circumscribe the domain of objects that can legitimately be considered under the rubric of "ethical debate." Terms like *euthanasia, confidentiality, autonomy and paternalism, genetic engineering,* and *in vitro fertilization* are not only well known today and easily employed in ordinary language but have come to be identified as the whole subject matter of medical ethics. At least in the field of medicine, an array of categories—which are exhaustively analyzed in the literature—has replaced the more humble, but less easily classifiable, process of grappling with ethical questions as they arise in the daily course of social life.[7] This testifies to the great power of the language and structure of bioethics, what we might call the "bioethical discourse," and the degree to which the assumption of the agenda of bioethics has in fact penetrated everyday life.

The limiting effects of the bioethical discourse in fact go further than this. They determine not just what is considered the appropriate domain of ethical argument but also the general strategy of argument itself. A question to be analyzed from the point of view of its ethical content is usually posed as a dilemma—that is, as a problem in a well-demarcated theoretical field which itself specifies the possible form of the solution. Thus, most commonly, it is postulated that particular choices need to be made from a narrow range of formal possibilities, each of which is associated with both attractive and unattractive implications. The discourse itself is subsequently directed toward guiding our choices and thereby supposedly resolving the dilemma. The effect of this procedure is that the focus is not on the actual process of clinical judgment but on formalized and abstracted representations of medical practice. Its validity, and indeed the validity of the criteria of judgment that are incorporated within it, is not subject to critical scrutiny from within the discipline of bioethics; nor could it be, for these criteria are, after all, the conditions of existence of the discourse itself.

For medical ethics, then, not only have the objects of study been circumscribed by the contemporary bioethical discourse but also the methods employed to study them have been limited. As a result, in respect of at least one aspect of its putative agenda, bioethics has already failed. Instead of opening up practical medicine to the critical instruments of the philosophical tradition, it has imposed a new, limited regime of its own. Instead of achieving an integration between the clinical disciplines and the cultural ones, it has widened the gulf. In the sense that will be explicated below, the practices of working doctors and the philosophical reflection on medicine are further apart than ever.

The underlying problem can be simply stated. The conventional approaches of medical ethics deviate fundamentally from the experiences of everyday medical practice. They are based on a mistaken notion of what medicine is about, a misunderstanding of both the ways in which ethical problems arise at the level of the clinic and the manner in which decisions are taken. The theoretical understanding of medicine, in other words, has to an important extent lost contact with the world of experience it was intended to represent. This is why the discipline itself has a very limited amount to offer practicing doctors or their patients.

The major concerns expressed in the public debates about medical ethics ignore many of the most important issues. They ignore, for example, the finely textured and subtle nature of the interaction between doctor and patient and the social context in which it occurs. They ignore the manner in which problems are formulated within this relationship and the ways in which the various possible courses of action are identified. Most importantly, they ignore the delicate ongoing process of negotiation and compromise that characterizes human relationships in general and in particular underlies any therapeutic interaction. Put differently, conventional medical ethics is unable to provide an understanding of, and hence a basis for intervention in, the medical lifeworld.

It may be observed that some of these claims can be interpreted in empirical terms and so ought to be able to be subjected to empirical scrutiny. Not surprisingly, evidence of this kind is presently difficult to obtain. However, of probably greater relevance is the converse empirical issue: there appears to have been no study showing that bioethical theory has produced a beneficial impact on medical decision making, or indeed, even that it has produced valuable effects in other ways for working doctors or their patients; the absence of such a study in itself may be taken to be of significance.[8]

It is appropriate to emphasize once more at this point that what is being considered here is the mainstream of contemporary bioethics, which comprises a vast body of literature with many contending themes and differences in emphasis. I am not suggesting that no analyses have been undertaken of the internal structure of the medical interaction; on the contrary, outstanding contributions have been made to our understanding of this relationship, as has already been mentioned and will be discussed further here.[9] Moreover, there is no intention to imply that the kinds of dilemmas considered in discussions about medical ethics do not occasionally arise or that the arguments that are employed there are completely irrelevant; indeed, the results of the arguments in the bioethical literature can be both interesting and valuable. However, from the point of view of their potential contribution toward the facilitation or enhancement of actual clinical practice, it must be recognized that such reflections are at best only partial. The vast majority of medical decisions are taken in an ethical environment in the absence of any obvious dilemma. They are made within an organic, ongoing relationship, in the spirit of open dialogue between doctor and patient. Accordingly, medical ethics needs to focus on the practical decision-making context. It must certainly be multidisciplinary—sociological, philosophical, psychological, and biological. More importantly, it needs to return to the real roots of medicine itself and to immerse itself in its own proper theoretical objects.

Microethics

Ethical questions in everyday clinical medicine are both more pervasive and more limited than the conventional perspective provided by bioethics would suggest. Crucial ethical issues are involved not just in the great questions of life and death but also in those clinical decisions which at first sight appear to be the simplest and most straightforward. It should be clear here that I am employing a very broad, although historically well-founded, notion of the nature of ethics.

This notion is encompassed within the classical Kantian formulation of the task of ethics and is especially appropriate for medicine. From the very first contact between doctor and patient to the last interaction that occurs between them, the ethical question, *"What should I do?",* is perpetually and critically at issue. This process includes every aspect of the communicative interaction. It includes the establishment of the implicit goals of the encounter and the taking of the history. It includes the conduct of the physical examination—in itself an extraordinary admixture of ethical and epistemological contents. It includes the choices made in deciding what investigations are to be undertaken and in formulating therapeutic strategies. Ethical decisions are implicated when the meanings of the outcomes are assessed and the community's possible interests in them are considered. In other words, medical ethics is not just about the dramatic questions that are discussed widely in the popular media or in the philosophical texts. *Ethics is what happens in every interaction between every doctor and every patient.*

The doctor is involved in a constant stream of choices of an ethical kind, which are made at the local level of his or her interaction with the patient and which bear on its most minute aspects. The accumulation of these "microethical" decisions, together with the technical decisions with which they are intimately linked, contributes importantly to the final outcome of any particular medical encounter. Arguably—allowing for the context in which the original approach to the doctor is made—medical outcomes depend more on the microethical decisions than on any other factors, including the decisions that may, in relevant circumstances, eventually emerge regarding the more familiar life and death issues. Yet the microethical environment of medicine is rarely discussed in medical courses from the point of view of its constitutive ethical nature;[10] it is virtually never considered in the international bioethics literature or popular debates.

In the clinical interaction, both doctor and patient are engaged in an unbroken continuum of ethical decision making. For the physician, there is a manner in which questions are asked of the patient and responses are made to the latter's answers or statements. This includes not only the choice of words but also the manner of their delivery: the tone of the voice, facial expressions, and so on. In addition, there is the degree of interest and compassion demonstrated when the more intimate matters are discussed.[11] During the physical examination, there is the general bearing that the doctor adopts and, in particular, the way in which those parts of it in which the patient might feel most vulnerable are conducted. Here, small matters may be very important: the time taken, the communication of commitment and concern, the sensitivity of the touch. The microethical context also embraces the kind of information given to the patient and the manner in which it is expressed. It includes the way in which the patient's participation in the decision-making process is obtained and the physician's openness to the contributions or suggestions that he or she might make. It includes the formulation of the problem and the decisions that are taken—regarding further investigation, therapy, or other strategies—to deal with it. And this is only the beginning. Every aspect of the relationship between doctor and patient is suffused with ethical considerations. Clinical medicine is immanently ethical; within it, the process of ethical judgment is continuous.

As far as the patient is concerned, a very similar situation exists. Here, too, a continuous flow of ethical decisions must be taken. These depend on the relationship established with the doctor, and they bear mainly on the conditions of the interaction itself. They determine, for example, the degree of openness to the doctor that is adopted, the kind of information that is offered, and the detail that is included; they determine the receptiveness to suggestions that might be made regarding underlying causes or lifestyle factors that might be considered contributory; and they determine the readiness to participate in any proposed therapeutic process.

In case this is thought to be insufficiently concrete, we can consider almost any actual interaction between a doctor and a patient. We may take as an example a perfectly mundane case of a young woman who attended an outpatient clinic complaining of nonspecific symptoms of tiredness and malaise over a protracted period. Here, as usual, a history needed to be taken; a physical examination needed to be conducted; and decisions about investigations, the diagnosis, and therapeutic strategies had to be made. At every point in the conversation between doctor and patient—which included the history—it was necessary to consider delicate and subtle issues regarding the way in which questions were asked or information was sought. How does one gain the trust of a person one has never met before, for example, to such an extent that she will grant access to her most private experiences? How should you ask about the effects of her illness? How should you broach the subject of any specific fears or anxieties she may have had? How do you ask about her sexual history and about contact with drugs or other infective sources? And what about the physical examination? How should you palpate the abdomen of someone who is frightened or anxious? How should you perform a gynecological examination—

which may in itself be painful or frightening or, for some women, be associated with unpleasant or even distressing connotations? These are all ethical questions that can be answered only when supplemented with the details of the practical discourse that is constituted by the actual interaction. They concern the ways in which we conduct ourselves at the actual point where clinical medicine is realized. They are, indeed, the real material of medical practice.[12] To be sure, the microethical issues are less dramatic than the more familiar bioethical concerns about the possible cessation of life-supporting treatments or the number of cells at which human life begins. Furthermore, from the point of view of many professional ethicists, these issues may lack philosophical interest or even "ethical significance," and they are difficult to formulate in terms of established, well-defined ethical categories or dilemmas demanding particular kinds of decisions. However—and this is the main point—the microethical considerations and their associated interactions are precisely what constitute the vast bulk of medical practice. More than any other factors, they determine the outcomes of actual clinical encounters. Indeed, clinical practice can only be properly understood and the problems that arise in medical decision making can only be adequately elucidated once the central and constitutive role of the microethical structure of medicine is recognized. Accordingly, its putative philosophical interest aside, in terms of relevance to the lives of ordinary people, microethics is of preeminent importance.[13]

Microethics is in general not the terrain of arresting cases involving heroic decisions or extraordinary circumstances arising at the extremes of medical practice; indeed, this may be one reason for the relative lack of attention it has attracted. Rather, it is the field of day-to-day communication and structured, complex interactions, of subtle gestures and fine nuances of language. Let us take another familiar example, this time of an elderly man who is anxiously awaiting the result of a biopsy of an abdominal mass that will show he has metastatic cancer. How should the biopsy information be conveyed to him? Here, the patient will invest every gesture and every intonation of the voice of the physician with weighty implications. The event itself will live with him, and during the course of his illness he will often return to it in his memory; no subsequent medical intervention will have such a powerful impact or such enduring consequences. The quality of his life, or what remains of it, and the decisions that he will make may well be determined at this time. The beginning of the conversation is straightforward enough: the doctor must make an opening statement and await the response of the patient; he must then provide the latter with an opportunity to consider the information and to determine what else he wants to know, or wants to avoid knowing. What happens after this cannot be predicted: it will depend on the doctor, the patient, and their interaction. Many issues will arise. In what manner should the prognosis of the illness be discussed, for example, in response to the patient's direct inquiry? What if no such inquiry is made? Should the subject be raised in any case? What should be said about the pain, the discomfort, and the uncertainty that can now be awaited? How should the physician respond to the man's despair, or to his bravado, or to his forced attempts at joviality? In this brief consultation, an almost unlimited array of microethical issues is raised, each of which may carry enduring implications for the patient.

Management of a labor and delivery raises special microethical issues. Here, too, the quality of the experience may have long-standing consequences, this time for both the parents and the child. The attention and care paid to the preparation for the labor will be especially important; this will include detailed discussions about many aspects of the process and the parents', the doctor's, and the midwife's preferences regarding various possible courses of action that might need to be considered. The physical circumstances of the labor and delivery, including the kind of lighting that is used and the aural environment, may also be important, as may be the facilities available for use during labor. In the course of labor itself, the kinds of medical assessment that should be carried out and the manner in which they are employed need to be carefully examined. Communication of the results of the physical examinations; advice or suggestions regarding the activity of the woman, including the positions she might adopt; and the contributions of a partner may be very sensitive issues with powerful consequences. Similarly, the more narrowly "medical" interventions raise the possibility of an inappropriate—and possibly inadvertant—exercise of power by medical personnel in circumstances where the woman and her partner may be especially vulnerable. To take one particular possibility that might arise: suppose a perineal tear is threatened and an episiotomy is contemplated. What are the factors that need to be taken into account? How should they be explained to the laboring woman, in order to obtain her consent? If the decision is in fact made to perform the procedure, how should it be carried out? To be sure, the "medical indications" for episiotomy can be found in standard textbooks; however, the possible enduring effects of an insensitively executed medical intervention cannot: the consequences of the fractured intimacy of the moment, and of the invasion of a profound experience, heavy with meaning, by gowned and gloved technicians. Medical management of a labor and delivery, therefore, including even an apparently "routine" episiotomy, has a complex ethical substratum. The decisions that are made at this level, furthermore, may be of great importance for the outcomes; indeed, it is possible to say that, in some respects at least, their importance may exceed that of the narrowly defined technical results.

Finally, consider a third-year medical student in an anesthesiology department who falsely gives a patient the impression that he is already a qualified doctor who is experienced in a technique he is about to apply.[14] It is easy to recognize here that telling a lie is wrong and to emphasize the importance of "informed consent." However, this may cover only part of the problem. As Eric Cassell has pointed out in an insightful commentary on this case, ethical issues such as truth-telling do not stand alone as timeless principles: they are important only "because of their place in human relations—of persons to themselves and to others."[15] Both the student and the patient are likely to be frightened and unsure; for this reason—and others—rather than being regarded as adversaries, the two should be seen as natural allies. Both have much to gain from the interaction and, indeed, the experience may be enriched by the student's openness and readiness to learn. The latter must set out actively to win the trust of the patient and to justify that trust with his actions. He will then come to understand that the medical interaction is a mutual one. On the doctor's part, furthermore, there are often doubts and uncertainties; for "that is the nature of medical care," of the "complex system of relationships and bonds that are part of the moral nature of the institution of medicine." This case shows how the established ethical categories may be revealed as partial and inadequate; by contrast, the microethical issues are broader and richer—and truer to the reality of clinical practice.[16]

The domain of ethical issues in medicine is much larger and more diverse than is generally accepted within the paradigms of conventional bioethics. What is often omitted by the latter is precisely an appreciation of the microethical context of clinical medicine and of the crucial role of this context in medical decision making. Although microethics may be more important for the determination of medical outcomes than most other factors, it is generally not considered in debates about medical ethics.

The consequences of this neglect of the microethical context of clinical medicine are substantial. Without an appreciation of the underlying structure of the reverberating physician-patient interaction, the nature of the medical relationship itself is obscured. The ethical decision-making process involving patient and doctor becomes profoundly distorted, seeming to be merely a matter of choosing, more or less arbitrarily, between alternatives rarely located in the real context of practical medicine and continuing interpersonal interaction. Communication between the participants becomes distorted or is never truly begun; this, in turn, leads to an exaggerated dependence on formal legal "solutions" to problems which ought to be resolved locally. In the worst case, it leads to the dismembering of clinical practice itself, with the responsibility for many qualitative judgments being passed to committees or, worse, to individuals who claim expertise not in a delimited area of knowledge, but in one ("bioethical") component of the complex—and intricate—process of medical decision making.[17]

It should now be clear how the microethical project differs from the bioethical one. Microethics starts from the premise that clinical practice consists of an accumulation of infinitesimal ethical events. Accordingly, its task is to chart the topography of the medical lifeworld, as it exists in its concreteness, its fluidity, and its temporal unpredictability. By this means, microethics seeks to reveal the structure and the dynamics of the clinical interaction and, in particular, to explicate the actual processes involved in clinical decision making. The bioethical formulation of the ethical content of medicine is quite different. It focuses on formal descriptions of dilemmas, which are themselves derived by a process of abstraction from the practical discursive context. These dilemmas, then, are representations of clinical practice within a pregiven theoretical framework; to these representations the methods and techniques of the theoretical system are subsequently applied.

Bioethics and microethics thus differ both in epistemological terms and at the foundational level of the constitution of their objects. From the point of view of microethics, bioethics is therefore not false, or erroneous, in the sense of contradicting the facts. Rather, it is considered to exist at a different level of generality and to be addressing different theoretical tasks. It is not a concern of bioethics to seek to apprehend in detail the complexity of the medical quotidian; indeed, it is not capable of doing so. Conversely, microethics is not concerned primarily with the formal structure of ethical dilemmas, which it considers to be of limited relevance for actual clinical practice. It does not deny, of course, as has been stated before, that dilemmas do occur from time to time in real practice and that classical bioethical considerations may then to a degree be useful. However, it contends that, in these very cases, the occurrence of a dilemma in itself is often merely indicative of a deeper problem—namely, the breakdown of the communicative process between the participants—so that in these circumstances this ought to become the main issue. In any event, regardless of the formulation, a "microethical" solution—that is, one at the level of the actual interaction between doctor and patient—must ultimately always be found, so there is no means by which the microethical realization of discourse can be circumvented.

The theoretical basis of microethics: the clinic as the foundation of modern medicine

A descriptive analysis of medical practice reveals the importance of its ethical content. This, in turn, raises the question of the status of the microethical within the overall structure of discourse and action which constitutes modern medicine. We need to clarify this status in order to define the ethical parameters in more detail and so to guide actual choices. Such a clarification is also useful in other respects, in that it allows certain theoretical problems of medicine— concerning both structural issues and questions of knowledge—to be elucidated with some rigor.

I claim that microethics has a theoretical basis that is at least as secure as that of traditional bioethics; indeed, I believe that it is more secure, because it is founded on the clinical experience itself. More specifically, the foundation is in the communicative processes that emerge from the forms of interaction that characterize the medical relationship, in association with the wider community within which they are articulated.

No attempt will be made here to develop in detail the elements of this theoretical foundation. Instead, the discussion will be restricted to a few rudimentary and programmatic remarks. My aim is threefold: to indicate some of the rich and diverse resources on which a theory of microethics can call and so to establish lines of continuity between microethics and existing projects, to sketch some preliminary conclusions from the present deliberations, and to identify some problems for future consideration.

Social relationships in general do not occur independently of each other, nor do they subsist in isolation from other forms of social life. Every relationship exists within a system of discourse that circumscribes its communicative possibilities and sets out rules of behavior. In other words, social life is partitioned into intersecting regions (or *language games,* to use a term that will be elaborated next), which form integrated systems of discourse and action. Each region has its own systematic structure that determines its characteristic modes of communication and the associated forms of social action. The medical relationship is one example of such an integrated system of discourse and action, with its particular structures that can be described in more or less precise detail. Furthermore, it carries a special interest because of the fundamental constitutive role it plays within medicine in general.

The medical interaction has a complex and dynamic structure that develops from a number of disparate sources. The description of this structure is as yet incomplete. We are able to say, however, that several levels are important. First, what might be called a level of *universal* structural determinants embraces the structures common to all instances of communication and their associated normative imperatives. These have been studied under the general heading of *universal pragmatics* or, more specifically, *discourse ethics* by Karl-Otto Apel, Jürgen Habermas, and others.[18] It also encompasses the historically determined central and formative role of the clinic in modern medicine, which has been described in detail by Michel Foucault and others, who have emphasized the importance of the changing nature of the relationship between doctor and patient in the history of medicine. The modern clinic, it must be said at once, is not a homogeneous entity; it has a complex structure which has yet to be fully elaborated.

At the highest possible level of generality, any interaction that has ethical content must take for granted certain assumptions—about the nature of communication, for example; about the rules of argumentation; and about the possibility that the various participants will change their attitudes or beliefs as a direct result of the interchange itself. If these presuppositions cannot be vindicated in real-life situations, moral judgments or behavior will no longer be possible. Apel and Habermas have set themselves the task of explicating the logical structure of this ethical substratum of all communicative interactions. Utilizing the strategy of a phenomenological description of the moral domain, they have sought to uncover the normative premises implicit in the acts that characterize the process of communication itself. The project is explicitly a Kantian one in that its concern is with the transcendental conditions of possibility of discourse—or even, of "normativity"; indeed, the "principle of universalization" that emerges from it bears a clear and explicit relationship to the categorical imperative.[19] Nonetheless, it does make a substantial new departure, to the extent that it shifts the focus of ethical reflection back to the social and intersubjective engagements that constitute communicative processes.

There can be no doubt that at the basis of every medical interaction there are certain fundamental assumptions about social behavior and ethical intercourse; furthermore, these undoubtedly are of great importance for the derivation of rules of ethical conduct within medicine. However—and this is readily accepted by Habermas himself[20]—these assumptions manifest themselves only in relation to the specific conditions of the particular practical discourse that characterizes medicine. Similarly, universal, transcendentally grounded rules of conduct within medicine become meaningful there only when considered in relation to the real horizon of the medical lifeworld. For this reason, the identification of these rules and structures is intimately linked to the explication of the characteristic discursive landscape of the clinical encounter.

It is now well recognized that the advent of modern medicine consisted largely of the formation of the clinic—or, more precisely, the development of the clinical encounter—as the practical locus of both knowledge and action.[21] Pre-modern medicine relied on a variety of therapeutic and interpretative techniques derived from a number of sources; these were only loosely and informally related to the physician-patient interaction, and they lacked a basis in a rigorous theory of the body. Development of the clinic introduced a set of highly disciplined procedures for both observing the body and obtaining information. Of course, there were very complex conceptual transformations presupposed in the development and refinement of this "clinical gaze." Furthermore, the clinic itself assumed an ambivalence that has ever since been both productive and limiting: on the one hand, there was the "scientific" reduction of disease and physical processes, which enabled the body to be opened up to systematic, empirical investigation; on the other, there was the ancient appreciation of the delicacy and mystery of embodied subjectivity and of the altered forms it assumes under conditions of illness. The former aspect derives, in the modern period, from the writings of Claude Bernard and his followers and has received much of the attention of historians of medicine (including Foucault). The latter can be traced back to the Hippocratic corpus; it has perdured alongside, and sometimes in opposition to, the scientific view. Its intellectual resources are different: within the clinical literature, Thomas Sydenham may be regarded as a notable advocate;[22] in contemporary times the theory of embodiment has been developed in detail by a number of authors.[23]

The two great themes of the scientific and the existential accounts of disease stand together in the contemporary clinic in an uneasy tension. Indeed, this tension has become one of the distinguishing marks of modern medicine and is the source both of its extraordinary heterogeneity and the unquenchable public fascination it arouses. Of greater relevance for our present purposes than the difference between these two aspects, however, is the common ground they share, which has made some compromise between them possible. Both recognize the special role of the clinic—that is, the potential potency of the interaction between patient and doctor, sufferer and skilled interpreter. As different as their premises are, both perspectives accept that this relationship is the principle source of medical knowledge of disease and disease processes. Accordingly, for both, the clinical encounter is not just a forum for the exchange of information between two individuals; it is a sophisticated epistemological tool which enables all the potential sources of knowledge about the patient and his or her illness to be effectively mobilized. Within it, as the structured, theoretical representation of the illness known as the "history," the special knowledge of the patient is at last formally recognized and granted a legitimate status; this is placed alongside the knowledge deriving from the direct experience of the physician, now formalized into the "physical examination."[24]

The clinical encounter is a place where things are created and accomplished. It is where the implications of knowledge are tested and where therapeutic action is initiated and pursued. It has become the occasion for the realization of practical decisions and their subsequent adjustment, in light of both their real outcomes and the particular perspectives and value systems of the participating individuals.[25]

The relation between doctor and patient, therefore, emerges from the history of medicine as a highly refined system of discourse closely linked to specific forms of action. Like the other systems of discourse and action that constitute the remainder of social life, it has a pregiven internal structure and is linked to an accompanying set of behavioral injunctions. These injunctions may reflect, at least in part, the universal conditions of communicative interactions, as they manifest themselves through the particular, concrete forms of the clinic. They impose, from within, a boundary on any given interaction; that is, the clinical interaction not only has internal structures but it is also governed by internal limits.

Sources of complexity in the doctor-patient relationship

It is important to realize, however, that these "universal" constraints are by no means the only ones to which the doctor-patient relationship is subjected. There is another, critically important, set of structural determinants: the value systems of the individuals involved. On the face of it, this seems straightforward: simply, each person enters the medical encounter with a given, preexisting set of values and value preferences. In reality, however, the advent of such systems of values is itself an extremely complex and difficult matter. This process has been studied in some detail;[26] in the present context it is sufficient to note merely that values are neither completely arbitrary nor fully determined. They are *contingent*, yet at the same time subject to constraints linked to the social configuration within which they are to be realized. They are themselves the outcomes of decisions and choices. It is worth saying further that, while choices need to be made, in the modern world the range of available possibilities is very great; indeed, it is clearly qualitatively greater than in any other epoch.[27]

Once a relationship has been established, there is a need for an ongoing process of decision making regarding various aspects of its conduct. These decisions will be subject to both the internal constraints (including personal values) and the external ones (the social milieu) we have mentioned. With respect to the medical encounter, it can be seen that the internal structure of the interaction itself and its implicit rules of conduct go a long way toward organizing it in a functional sense. At the same time, the values of each participant further limit the realization of the institutional structures. The medical interaction, therefore, as we have mentioned before, has a complex and heterogeneous structure; it is precisely this complex structure which generates the microethical imperatives.

The modern person occupies many roles; more precisely, he or she participates in many of these integrated systems of discourse and action. For example, a physician is also a citizen, research worker, father or mother, teacher, or even political activist. Systems like this have been given the name *language games*, a term we shall employ here. The original idea derives from the work of Ludwig Wittgenstein, who used it to refer to the loose constellation of meanings that together constitute a concept. In the expanded context adopted here, it refers to the constellation of meanings that make up a particular sphere of activity of an individual; it is not restricted merely to concepts, but applies also to processes of communication and structures of behavior. The concept is useful because, by its emphasis on the unity of communicative discourse and social action, it enables us to identify and delimit various regions of social life that exist as integral forms and to analyze their internal structures; in other words, it enables us to recognize and understand in a systematic way particular types of behavior, relationships, or interactions.[28]

Language games may be highly heterogeneous, to the point that the goals and values potentially realizable within some of them may be in open conflict. Every person, however, learns to operate within the constraints of each relevant language game—that is, to follow the rules and to acquire facility with a variety of discourse systems. In each language game, furthermore, decisions about right conduct need to be made. The demands of some language games may be different from those of the others, as we have said. In addition, they may vary according to changing circumstances and, in particular, according to the ongoing interactions between subjects engaged in structured communication and dialogue within them.[29]

The decision-making process, therefore, is not without structure and is certainly not arbitrary. However, it has many degrees of freedom, and its variables may change more or less independently of each other. All of this is very clear in the case of the medical encounter. Interchanges between doctors and patients are extremely heterogeneous. There are certainly formal discursive regularities—that is to say, constant structural features of the clinical encounter which distinguish it from all other interactions. At the same time, however, there are major and often quite unpredictable variations. Individuals belong simultaneously to several—sometimes very many—domains of discourse and action, and each of these, as we have said, has its own grammar: its own rules of conduct and its own more or less complex forms of communication and knowledge. This heterogeneity and its accompanying complexity is in part a consequence of the pluralist nature of modern society which has led to a great proliferation of the language games to which a given individual belongs. This proliferation has proved both liberating and limiting, for it simultaneously provides both a greatly expanded context for action and imposes many new constraints on it. However this may be, each social role has associated with it ethical duties and obligations; it is not unexpected that from time to time some of these conflict.

It goes without saying that exactly the same considerations apply to the people who come to doctors as patients. Accordingly, to adopt the point of view of the doctor for the sake of illustration, in addition to their own highly variable roles, within the clinical encounter itself doctors are called on to interact with many different kinds of people, each of whom has a distinctive set of values and goals. For example, it would not be surprising for a doctor in a single afternoon to see a young, gay professional man, a middle-aged female migrant factory worker, and an elderly retired farmer who has taken off the entire day to make the trip down from the country. Such a range of interactions is of course in no way unfamiliar; however, it does indicate the versatility that is demanded of a practicing clinician: he or she is required to be engaged in a constant process of transcription and translation across systems of discourse. The process of communication must be able to be adapted to the specific settings that are appropriate for particular patients; we are all only too well aware of what happens when mistakes are made at this level.

Some consequences

The complex, multifaceted nature of the medical interaction is accessible to investigation with the help of a variety of well-established tools. These enable the structures of the medical lifeworld to be elucidated without loss of concreteness or specificity. The task is in part that of a phenomenological description of the experience of the clinic; however, it is not merely this, for it also requires an explication of a relationship that is structured and laden with ethical imperatives. The medical lifeworld is multifaceted and highly differentiated; it contains as one of its irreducible elements a form of intersubjectivity that is historically structured. Superimposed on the universal structures are historically and socially contingent variables.

The above considerations lead to a strong conclusion regarding medical relationships, one which has profound implications for ethical decision making. The interactions that occur in the medical encounter and the decisions that come out of them are not determinate. They are contingent, just as are the value systems that are superimposed on them. Their courses cannot be predicted, for they depend very sensitively, and unpredictably, not only on the precise factual details of the patient's illness but also on the course of the actual interchanges that occur between patient and physician.[30]

At the outset, the relationship is indeterminate: its course cannot be predicted. Accordingly, the cumulative outcome of a series of decisions may be very different from the decision that might have been made in retrospect with full knowledge of all of the circumstances that subsequently developed. Every clinician is familiar with this phenomenon: the result of a long series of decisions, each of which has been taken in good faith and after careful consideration, may be the very outcome which at the beginning seemed least desirable; to have avoided it, however, would have required the employment at some stage of unethical, or at least questionable, means.

There are no "typical cases" in clinical medicine from the point of view of ethics or communicative dialogue. Each "case" has its own irreducible particularity. Both parties enter the relationship with values, and with expectations, but without knowing what will be discovered and what will thus be created. This fundamental conclusion vitiates a large part of the contemporary discourse about "medical ethics"; it means also that there is no alternative to the microethical route.

An example may be helpful here which illustrates both the nature of clinical practice and the inadequacy of the bioethical perspective. A problem was set for an ethics class for medical students in the following terms:

A patient of yours, or one you have observed, is diagnosed as having a serious sexually transmitted disease. You later learn that the patient has just started a relationship with your best friend. What should you do?

At first glance, this formulation appears to be unremarkable. It is clear that it invites the students to consider whether they would favor releasing confidential information to a third person; the expected debate would be concerned with the value of confidentiality and its limitations, especially in relation to the principles of autonomy, nonmaleficence, beneficence, and justice, and possibly with the legal implications of both disclosure and nondisclosure.[31] *In the real situation,* however, what would occur is something very different. A process of discussion would be initiated between the doctor and the patient. In due course, the problem would be raised and the issues debated in as much detail as was necessary. Where the debate would end in the real case no one can say—and, indeed, no one ought to be able to say if human interactions are to retain meaningful content. An infinite array of outcomes is possible; some of these have desirable and some have undesirable implications. The question suggested in the bioethical formulation may not ultimately be the most important issue, or, indeed, it may even turn out not to be an issue at all: in fact, it is extremely uncommon for a patient to refuse to tell a friend or relative about a possible medical risk. Instead, what may emerge as most important may be, for example, the patient's own concerns about his or her body; it may be the fear of illness or even death; it may be anxiety about a particular relationship or about relationships in general; or it may involve concern about apparently extraneous matters like employment or financial security. These considerations may seem to be begging the question of ethical debate; nonetheless, they are precisely the ones that predominate in clinical work. In clinical interactions all we can do is to say where we will start and how we will proceed; the rest—subject to the requirements of microethical structures—is up to the interchange itself.

Conclusion and directions for future research

The principal concern of this essay has been the practical business of medical decision making. We have seen how in the flow of clinical interaction a continuum of decisions of almost infinitesimal magnitude arises. Each decision has a small but finite ethical content; their cumulative sum determines both the qualitative and the quantitative outcomes of the medical encounter.

This microethical level is not merely incidental to medicine; on the contrary, it is actually the crux of it. Clinical practice proceeds exactly by such local, piecemeal mechanisms. At the outset of most clinical relationships the overall outcomes are largely indeterminate. What also must be borne in mind is that the proliferation of the language games in which the individuals in modern society participate has substantially increased the possibilities for conflict within the medical interaction.

These results are basic facts of modern medicine which must now be accepted by anyone—doctor or patient—who participates in it. They emphasize the contingency of clinical medicine, but also its great richness and complexity. What is more, they indicate the direction in which we must move if we are to deepen our understanding of the nature of medical decision making and thereby to preserve the vitality and the integrity of clinical medicine. The language game of contemporary bioethical discourse is too far removed from the real experience of the clinic to provide the insights and guidance that are required to respond to the concerns of the community about the way in which medicine has developed; this is a task only a return to the microethical level can accomplish.

The return to the microethical world of medicine will mean several things. It will mean the explicit reestablishment of the clinical relationship at the center of medicine. It will mean the careful elucidation and renewed understanding of the structures of this relationship. But it will also mean the opening of new and potentially productive research projects. The many problems that immediately suggest themselves with the formulation of the issues in terms of microethics may lead to fertile areas of research. One question, for example, concerns the relationship between microethical and "macroethical" levels of action.[32] In particular, the status of the systems of philosophical ethics that command such attention today—such as utilitarianism and "deontology"—will require clarification from the new perspective. Second, there is the question of the details of the substructure of the microethical context, especially in light of changing economic and technical conditions of medical practice; here, much work is needed to identify the ethical residues at the core of microethical discourse and the foundational imperatives that arise with them.[33] Third, there is the perpetual but nonetheless critical boundary problem: the problem of what to do at the limits of microethical discourse, when, for example, one of the participants to the relationship refuses to act in an ethical manner. None of the extant philosophical perspectives provides a satisfactory solution to this problem; however, examination of the nature of systems of discourse in a larger context, as suggested by the microethical approach, may provide some new strategies for construction of a pathology of the ethical relationship.[34] Finally, there is a whole series of fundamental questions at the epistemological level which need to be considered, including questions concerning the place of science within medicine and in relation to the medical interaction.[35]

For all these reasons, it is time for the central importance of the microethical aspect of medicine to be recognized and for it to be established as a major area of study in its own right. We must not allow ethical debate in medicine to be restricted to discussions about embryo experimentation or life support systems, to the neglect of the actual, vital decisions that characterize our everyday work. Let us instead return to the living, ethical core of medicine—both as it is and as it ought to be.

Notes

1   See, for example, I. Illich, *Limits to Medicine* (London, Marion Boyars, 1977); R. Taylor, *Medicine out of Control* (Melbourne, Sun Books, 1979); G. Corea, *The Mother Machine: From Artificial Insemination to Artificial Wombs* (New York, Harper and Row, 1985).

2   R. L. Holmes, "The Limited Relevance of Analytical Ethics to the Problems of Bioethics," *Journal of Medicine and Philosophy* 15 (1990): 143–160; B. A. Brody, "Quality of Scholarship in Bioethics," *Journal of Medicine and Philosophy* 15 (1990): 161–178.

3   M. Siegler, "Clinical Ethics and Clinical Medicine," *Archives of Internal Medicine* 139 (1979): 914–915; C. D. Clements, "Bioethical Essentialism and Scientific Population Thinking." *Perspectives in Biology and Medicine* 28 (1985): 188–207; E. J. Cassell, *The Healer's Art: A New Approach to the Doctor-Patient Relationship* (Philadelphia, Lippincott, 1976).

4   R. M. Zaner, *Ethics and the Clinical Encounter* (Englewood Cliffs, N.J.; Prentice-Hall, 1988); R. C. Fox, "Evolution of American Bioethics: A Sociological Perspective," in G. Weisz, ed., *Social Science Perspectives on Medical Ethics* (Amsterdam, Kluwer, 1990), pp. 201–217.

5   A. MacIntyre, *After Virtue: A Study in Moral Theory* (London, Duckworth, 1987); B. Williams, *Ethics and the Limits of Philosophy* (London, Fontana, 1985); C. Taylor, *Sources of the Self: The Making of the Modern Identity* (Cambridge, Harvard University Press, 1989); see also M. Charlesworth, "Bioethics and the Limits of Philosophy," *Bioethics News* 9 (1989): 1–24; C. Gilligan, *In a Different Voice: Psychological Theory and Women's Development* (Cambridge, Harvard University Press, 1982).

6   See Seigler, "Clinical Ethics."

7   The literature of bioethics is very extensive and sophisticated. Among the best-known and

most celebrated texts are the following: T. L. Beauchamp and J. F. Childress, *Principles of Biomedical Ethics* (New York, Oxford University Press, 1983); T. L. Beauchamp and L. Walters, eds., *Contemporary Issues in Bioethics* (Belmont, Calif., Wadsworth, 1982); R. M. Veatch, *A Theory of Medical Ethics* (New York, Basic Books, 1981); J. Glover, *Causing Death and Saving Lives* (New York, Penguin, 1977); P. Singer, *Practical Ethics* (Cambridge, Cambridge University Press, 1979); T. L. Regan, ed., *Matters of Life and Death: New Introductory Essays in Moral Philosophy* (New York, Random House, 1980). As this list indicates, bioethics is a heterogeneous area of thought encompassing diverse themes; further, it should be noted that not all the work of individual authors who operate within the bioethical paradigms necessarily falls inside it.

8   See note 13 below.

9   E. D. Pellegrino, and D. C. Thomasma, *A Philosophical Basis of Medical Practice* (New York, Oxford University Press, 1981); Zaner, *Ethics and the Clinical Encounter*; D. Crane, *The Sanctity of Social Life: Physicians' Treatment of Critically Ill Patients* (New York, Russell Sage, 1975); J. Ladd, "The Internal Morality of Medicine: An Essential Dimension of the Patient-Physician Relationship," in E. A. Shelp, ed., *The Clinical Encounter: The Moral Fabric of the Physician-Patient Relationship* (Dordrecht, Reidel, 1983), pp. 209–231.

10   The major reports that have considered in detail the questions associated with ethics teaching in medical courses have not considered the microethical issues. See P. A. Komesaroff, "The Nature of Medicine and the Teaching of Medical Ethics," *Bioethics* 4(1990): 66–77.

11   Cf. E. J. Cassell, *Talking with Patients* (Cambridge, MIT Press, 1985).

12   Cf. J. La Puma and D. L. Schiedermayer, "The Clinical Ethicist at the Bedside," *Theoretical Medicine* 12(1991): 141–149; and D. S. Davis, "Rich Cases: The Ethics of Thick Description," *Hastings Center Report* 21(1991): 12–16. See also C. M. Culver, ed., *Ethics at the Bedside* (London, University Press of New England, 1990).

13   Although, as mentioned, evidence for the clinical utility of bioethics is lacking, in relation to the microethical variables such evidence abounds. For example, one method of studying the outcomes of clinical medicine is to examine "patient satisfaction"; here, the evidence points strongly in favor of microethics. See, e.g., J. A. Hall and M. C. Dornan, "What Patients Like about Their Medical Care and How Often They Are Asked: A Meta-analysis of the Satisfaction Literature," *Social Science in Medicine* 27(1988): 935–939; B. S. Hulka, L. L. Kupper, J. C. Cassel, and R. A. Babineau, "Practice Characteristics and Quality of Primary Medical Care: The Doctor-Patient Relationship," *Medical Care* 13 (1975): 808–820.

14   M. D. Basson, "The 'Student Doctor' and a Wary Patient," and E. J. Cassel, "Commentary," both in C. Levine and R. M. Veatch, eds., *Cases in Bioethics* (New York, Hastings Center, 1984), pp. 26–27.

15   Cassel, "Commentary," p. 27.

16   For additional examples, see Zaner, *Ethics and the Clinical Encounter*, and Cassell, *Talking with Patients*.

17   The practice of "bioethics consultancies" has grown in recent years; see, e.g., "Bioethics Consultation: American Style," *Bulletin of Medical Ethics* (May 1990): 5. While it is important that clinical practice is not dismembered, this does not exclude the possibility of fruitful contributions from sources outside the therapeutic relationship; see, e.g., Zaner, *Ethics and the*

Clinical Encounter, and J. D. Moreno, "Ethics Consultation as Moral Engagement," *Bioethics* 5(1991): 44–56.

18 See, for example, J. Habermas, *Moral Consciousness and Communicative Action* (Cambridge, MIT Press, 1990); K-O. Apel, *Towards the Transformation of Philosophy* (London, Routledge and Kegan Paul, 1980); S. Benhabib and F. Dallmayr, eds., *The Communicative Ethics Controversy* (Cambridge, MIT Press, 1990); D. Rasmussen, ed., *Universalism vs. Communitarianism: Contemporary Debates in Ethics* (Cambridge, MIT Press, 1990).

19 J. Habermas, "Discourse Ethics: Notes on a Programme of Philosophical Justification," in Benhabib and Dallmayr, *Communicative Ethics Controversy,* p. 90.

20 Ibid., pp. 100–101.

21 M. Foucault, *The Birth of the Clinic* (London, Tavistock, 1973). See also Pellegrino and Thomasma, *Philosophical Basis of Medical Practice,* and E. J. Pellegrino, "The Healing Relationship: The Architechtonics of Clinical Medicine," in Shelp, *Clinical Encounter,* pp. 153–172; M. C. Rawlinson, "Foucault's Strategy: Knowledge, Power and the Specificity of Truth." *Journal of Medicine and Philosophy* 12(1987): 371–396.

22 It is claimed by Engelhardt that, by "(bracketing) philosophical and scientific presuppositions" in order to "describe the presented reality of patient's illnesses," Sydenham sought to develop "an eidetic phenomenology of disease." See H. T. Engelhardt, Jr., "Illnesses, Diseases and Sicknesses," in V. Kestenbaum, ed., *The Humanity of the Ill: Phenomenological Perspectives* (Knoxville, University of Tennessee Press, 1982), pp. 142–157.

23 See M. Merleau-Ponty, *The Phenomenology of Perception* (London, Routledge and Kegan Paul, 1960); P. Ricoeur, *Freedom and Nature: The Voluntary and the Involuntary* (Evanston, Ill., Northwestern University Press, 1966); see also R. M. Zaner, *The Problem of Embodiment* (The Hague, Martinus Nijhoff, 1971); Zaner, "Embodiment," in W. T. Reich, *The Encyclopedia of Bioethics* (London, Free Press, 1978), pp. 361–366; D. Leeder, "Medicine and Paradigms of Embodiment," *Journal of Medicine and Philosophy* 9(1989): 29–44; M. C. Rawlinson, "Medicine's Discourse and the Practice of Medicine," in Kestenbaum, *Humanity of the Ill,* pp. 69–85.

24 Cf. G. Canguilhem, *On the Normal and the Pathological* (Dordrecht, D. Reidel, 1978).

25 See V. Kestenbaum, ed., "Introduction: The Experience of Illness," in Kestenbaum, *Humanity of the Ill,* pp. 3–39 and other essays in this volume; and R. M. Zaner, *The Context of Self* (Athens, Ohio University Press, 1981).

26 L. Kohlberg, *The Philosophy of Moral Development: Moral Stages and the Idea of Justice* (San Francisco, Harper and Row, 1981); J. Piaget, *The Moral Judgement of the Child* (London, Routledge and Kegan Paul, 1965); Habermas, *Moral Consciousness and Communicative Action;* see also Gilligan, *In a Different Voice.*

27 A. Heller, *A Philosophy of Morals* (London, Blackwell, 1990), chaps. 1 and 4.

28 L. Wittgenstein, *Philosophical Investigations,* trans. G. E. M. Anscombe, (Oxford, Blackwell, 1974); Apel, K-O. Op. cit., chapter 1; cf. also R. Sokolowski, "The Art and Science of Medicine," in Pellegrino et al., *Catholic Perspectives on Medical Morals,* pp. 263–275. Other formulations of related ideas may be found in the works of other authors; for example, "finite provinces of meaning" (Schutz) or "social practices" (MacIntyre). The concept of "language game" is also employed, albeit with a somewhat different content, by J-F. Lyotard, *The Postmodern Condition: A Report on Knowledge* (Manchester, Manchester University Press, 1986).

29   See also G. Skirbekk, "Contextual and Universal Pragmatics: Mutual Criticism of Praxeologi-
       cal and Transcendental Pragmatics," Ph.D. Thesis 11 28(1991): 35–51, and R. Sokolowski, "The
       Art and Science of Medicine," in Pellegrino, et al., *Catholic Perspectives on Medical Morals,*
       pp. 263–275.

30   Cf. M. Weber, "Politics as a Vocation," in H. H. Gerth and C. W. Mills, eds., *From Max Weber*
       (London, Routledge and Kegan Paul, 1948), pp. 77–128; Zaner, *Ethics and the Clinical Encoun-
       ter,* chap. 1.

31   See, e.g., L. Walters, "Ethical Aspects of Medical Confidentiality," in T. L. Beauchamp and
       L. Walters, eds., *Contemporary Issues in Bioethics* (San Francisco, Wadsworth, 1978), pp. 169–
       175; R. Gillon, "AIDS and Medical Confidentiality," *British Medical Journal* 294(1987): 1675–
       1677; A. Orr, "Legal AIDS: Implications of AIDS for British and American Law," *Journal of
       Medical Ethics* 15(1989): 161–167.

32   R. Sokolowski, *Moral Action: A Phenomenological View* (Bloomington, Indiana University
       Press, 1985).

33   J. Habermas, *Theory of Communicative Action,* 2 vols., trans. T. McCarthy (Boston, Beacon,
       1984/7); H. Jonas, *The Imperative of Responsibility: In Search of an Ethics for the Technological
       Age* (Chicago: Chicago University Press, 1984).

34   Cf. B. Williams, *Moral Luck* (Cambridge, Cambridge University Press, 1988), chap. 5; Haber-
       mas, "Discourse Ethics," pp. 79–95; Zaner, *Ethics and the Clinical Encounter,* pp. 255–258.

35   P. A. Komesaroff, *Objectivity, Science and Society* (London, Routledge and Kegan Paul, 1986);
       see also A. MacIntyre, "Objectivity in Morality and Objectivity in Science," in H. T. Engel-
       hardt, Jr. and D. Callahan, eds., *Morals, Science and Sociality* (New York, Hastings Center,
       1978), pp. 21–39.

Science, medicine, and illness: rediscovering the patient as a person

Paul Redding

In the twentieth century the progressive application of the experimental sciences to the practice of medicine has endowed it with powers unimagined in earlier times. But, it is commonly complained, this has been achieved at a price—that of the "depersonalization" of the healing experience. Should this be seen as an inevitable effect of the increasing penetration of science into the healer's art? How should practitioners and patients address this problem? These are questions as difficult to answer as they are important to ask. We might start to address them by first attempting to understand something about what happens when everyday knowledge, the sort of knowledge possessed by all cultures, becomes science—the sort of knowledge which for the most part has been the achievement of modern European culture alone.

"Observing with their own eyes": the problem of objectivity

We might look to the Copernican revolution standing at the threshold of the age of modern science as exemplifying a characteristically modern distrust, fueled by scientific discovery, of the way the world is given in immediate everyday experience. Once historians used to portray such scientific breakthroughs as resulting from a reawakening of interest in the observable world. In contrast to their medieval predecessors, early modern scientists, so the story went, turned from their books and theoretical controversies to the world itself in order to learn its secrets. More recent philosophers of science, however, have shown this story to be largely mythical.[1] It is now commonly argued that the "bookish" Aristotelian science of the Middle Ages was, in comparison to the science that replaced it, just as adequate to the world of simple observation. In fact, in its struggle with the classical Aristotelian cosmology, the emerging modern physics was in many ways in apparent conflict with the experienced world and had to employ abstract theoretical arguments to first cast doubt upon and then reinterpret that experience.[2]

One aspect of this involved interpreting some particular, previously unproblematic, experience as revealing an only "apparent" rather than real state of affairs. Copernicus himself did this by inquiring into the nature of the conditions under which the experience of the movement of the stars and planets occurred. While the pre-Copernicans believed what they observed with their own eyes—the daily passage of the sun around the earth—Copernicus asked whether it might not be the case that rather than the *observer* being at rest it was the sun, while the observer observed from the surface of a diurnally rotating earth. With this postulation the earlier *real* movement of the sun had now become *merely apparent,* as had the observer's earlier repose.

Copernicus' move here, a move that was to become typical of much subsequent scientific thought, "denaturalizes" experience and, in directing attention to a variety of possible conditions, problematizes and relativizes it. The original observer is now seen as having viewed the world uncritically from *a particular place in it*: as the experience was from a particular point of view or perspective, the content of experience must be reinterpreted as relative to that perspective.[3]

In fact, this maneuver of thought could be, and was, taken further. The idea of particular *conditions* of experience could be extended, metaphorically as it were, internally to the characteristic make up of the experiencing subject as well. In this way, both Descartes and Galileo revived an ancient philosophical distinction—that between the "primary" qualities of extension and shape and the "secondary" ones such as color or smell.[4]

This distinction further problematized the everyday world because only the former were thought of as really belonging to the world itself. The secondary qualities, it was thought, only *appeared* to belong to the world itself: in reality they were "subjective" and, like "feelings," were located in the mind rather than the world. With this, the real world became thought of as only open to the highly abstract gaze of the theoretical scientist; in contrast, the everyday world became an error.

In modern scientific medicine, an analogous distinction between the "subjective" and scientific (or objective) views of an illness is found in the distinction between the perspectives of patient and doctor. The patient knows the disease from the point of view of his or her own lived body. He or she knows what it is like to be sick and gives expression to this view in recounting the symptoms. From the doctor's theoretically grounded diagnostic and therapeutic perspective, however, the specific complaints of the patient are downgraded as forms of knowledge. They reveal only the perspectival and subjective "appearance" of the problem—that of the "underlying" disease to be understood theoretically.

In this way the original symptoms recounted by the patient lose their status as *claims* made by an intentional speaking subject about some reality. Like the diagnostic "signs" detected in the physical examination and like the results of further investigative procedures, they are now interpreted as *effects* of underlying pathological processes about which the patient is fundamentally ignorant. The truth of this process will only be revealed when it is no longer seen from the first-person point of view of the patient but reinterpreted into the language of the models and theories, experimental procedures, and statistical correlations of medical science.

This characteristic of modern medical science is a consequence of the fact that it, like the paradigm modern science, physics, emerged in a series of complex ruptures from the "life-world" of everyday experienced reality. Once modern physics had claimed its abstract, mathematizable structures as the reality beyond the erroneous appearances of experience, the mechanistic conceptions and schemata used to explain the movement of the planets and the trajectories of missiles would eventually be applied to the human body.

Already in the seventeenth century, close on the heels of the new physical discoveries, Descartes and Hobbes had put forward speculative mechanistic "physiologies" attempting to demonstrate human behaviour as the effects of complicated mechanical contrivances. And yet while the idea of mechanism consequent to the birth of physics may have been a prerequisite to the emergence of modern medical science, mechanics itself was not sufficient for that development. The establishment of a truly scientific physiology needed the conceptual rearticulation of the body as a mechanism that was brought about by the revolutionary thought of Claude Bernard in the nineteenth century. With his notion of a *milieu interieur*—the "internal environment" permeating the substance of the body as such—Bernard could develop a usable deterministic representation of the body, a representation able to be linked to experimental procedures and instrumental interventions. It was this sort of link that the cruder physics-based seventeenth- and eighteenth-century conceptions of mechanism had been unable to achieve.[5]

However, once achieved, this change in epistemological structure had the same effects with respect to the body that earlier physics had with respect to the physical world in general. The mechanistic physiologies of Descartes and Hobbes had really only amounted to expressions of faith in the mechanistic body: Bernard's revolutionary reinterpretation of the concept of mechanism vindicated that faith.

Scientific civilization and its discontents: some questions

The more recent views of the history of science, to which I have alluded, draw attention to the discontinuities within knowledge and postulate different styles of knowing; they also raise questions that were not easily raised by the earlier view which saw science as the mere accumulation of a single and homogeneous form of knowledge. It can easily be seen how this latter view could have gone along with a generally optimistic assessment of the role of science in the world: If knowledge is a good thing why is not more of it even better? But from the view which speaks of discontinuities and distinct forms of knowledge, more substantial questions arise. Is the wholesale replacement of one form of knowledge by another necessarily a good thing? Are there losses of knowledge as well as gains involved in those typical epistemological transformations characteristic of modernity?

While such questions have increased in recent times, in fact they date back almost as far as the scientific revolution itself.[6] In the early eighteenth century, for example, there appears to have been a widespread revival of earlier "humanistic" cultural forms in Europe in response to what was perceived as the ethically skeptical consequences of the new worldview. It seems to have been thought that the mechanical view of the world consequent on the new physics would threaten the ethical fabric of life by rendering subjective and merely apparent all ethical qualities. In retrospect, such a diagnosis seems percipient. It was essentially repeated in the late nineteenth century by Nietzsche under the description of nihilism. Later, the sociologist Max Weber characterized the modern world as having become "disenchanted" under the impact of modern science-based rationality. In the twentieth century numerous variations have been played on this theme by different cultural critics.[7]

Looked at from the point of view of the increasing dominance of a single type of rationality, the story of the development of modernity gains a very different gloss. In the earlier optimistic narrative the growth of science was told as the progressive illumination of the world allowing it to be seen in its glory. In the latter, however, it is told as the monopolization by a single mode of interpretation of the world, the progressive eclipse of rival views of the world by the imposition of a single epistemological regime.

Within the epistemology of modern science, knowledge has been conceived in a radically different way to the way in which it had been conceived in pre-modern times. It has also differed fundamentally from the conceptions of knowledge implicit within both everyday life and modern humanistic culture. The key notion in this new epistemology was *prediction*, as it was predictability of outcome that linked theoretical representation to experimental procedure and instrumental application. Hypothesized laws could be tested on the basis of their predictive power and, once established, could be applied in ways to bring about various predictable results. We might say that from the viewpoint of modern classical physics, to know is to be able to predict: the predictability at the center of experimental testing and technical application becomes the criterion for all genuine knowledge.

In medicine, as in modern culture at large, recently attention has started to swing more and more from the traditionally celebrated benefits of such an instrumental rationality to its increasingly obvious costs. As medicine has become increasingly "rationalized," the doctor has come to be seen by many as merging more and more into the role of "technoscientist"—a manipulator and regulator of complex natural systems. Such a technoscientist, armed with the powerful predictive knowledge that the medical sciences provide, is able to intervene into the operations of that particular system of systems which we otherwise know as a person: "otherwise" because from the point of view of the discourse and practice of such a technoscience, the object of such a practice can no longer simply be identified with what we know as a "person."

When we view the development of medicine in this way—that is, in terms of the increasingly central role played by the paradigm of instrumental reason—we will see complaints such as those concerning the increasing "depersonalization" of medical practice as indicators of underlying structural features of modern medical practice rather than as simply reflecting on the characters of its practitioners. Furthermore, from such a perspective we will see the questions involved in a confrontation with these issues as an aspect of that question which the hermeneutic philosopher Hans-Georg Gadamer has claimed as the central to the modern age: "The question of how our natural view of the world—the experience of the world that we have as we simply live our lives—is related to the unassailable and anonymous authority that confronts us in the pronouncements of science."[8] Indeed, the task confronting the tradition of medical practice in dealing with such issues will be an aspect of what Gadamer sees as the quintessential modern task: the task to "reconnect the objective world of technology, which the sciences place at our disposal and discretion, with those fundamental orders of our being that are never arbitrary or manipulable by us, but rather, simply demand our respect."[9]

Ethics of science, science of ethics

Medical culture has indeed started to reflect on the consequences of the awesome powers put at its disposal by modern medical science. Recent attention-grabbing developments within medical technologies, such as within the areas of in vitro fertilization and genetic engineering, have focused attention on the ethical issues surrounding medical practice and have spawned the specialist area of "bioethics." As welcome as such an engagement of philosophical reflection with medical practice may be, it can still be argued that the scope and depth of the dilemmas of modern medical practice typically tend to go unrecognized. First, concentration on such "big" ethical issues tends to leave the basic practices of medicine relatively untouched. From the perspective of the dilemmas of instrumental rationality, it is the ethical dimension of the structural depersonalization of the modern medical encounter under the impact of science that itself needs addressing. But another problem arises when it is the ethics side of the "bioethics" compound that is focused on.

It is perhaps not surprising that within the rhetoric of the engagement of "ethics" with medicine, ethics itself sometimes sounds like a branch of modern science—a discipline that is capable of being "applied" in concrete situations and which claims a particular place within the complex division of labor of the scientific edifice. One gains the impression of the professional "ethicist" as yet another specialist member of the modern medical "team": the philosophical analogue of the biophysicist or the micropathologist, there to bring their own "unassailable and anonymous authority" to bear on ethical questions associated with the application of medicotechnical power.

Indeed, in part such an image does come close to one way in which moral philosophy has itself imagined its own role in the world in the modern period. Philosophy, no less than medicine, was transformed in the early modern period under the impact of science, and we might see the existence of "moral philosophy" as such as consequent on the cultural changes brought about by the scientific revolution.

Introducing as they did a comprehensive secular version of the world, the modern sciences created a demand for a secular version of the ethical doctrines previously encoded within religion. But perhaps more seriously, the scientific worldview itself created an ethical crisis in its demolition of the world of everyday appearances. Within the pre-modern Aristotelian worldview the "objectivity" of evaluative qualities such as ethical and aesthetic ones could easily be accepted. With the ascendancy of the mathematizable world of physics, however, such ethical qualities went the way of the "secondary" qualities of color, smell, and taste: they were now construed as "subjective." Simply put, morality, like beauty, became removed from the world and placed "in the eye of the beholder." To counter such a threatening nihilistic ethical skepticism, a new science was necessary, the science of *morals*. The difficulty has been that, assessed on the model of modern science, ethics appears to have been a failure. While many have aspired to be the Newton, Lavoisier, or Bernard of the moral world, modern ethical philosophy has simply never been consolidated in a way analogous to the sciences.

It could be argued, of course, that we are now in a position with respect to an "objective" philosophical sciences of ethics that is analogous to that of pre-Bernardian medicine or pre-Copernican astronomy. Ethics just has to wait for its revolutionary theorist. But within recent philosophical ethics there has been a growing number of writers who see the whole problematic of anything like a modern "science" of morality as deeply flawed.[10] Such voices have something in common with those which, coming from a wider philosophical perspective, have questioned the self-conception, the functioning, and the structure of the whole modern philosophical problematic.[11] For these critics, the sorts of problems facing medical practice and those affecting philosophy are of the same kind. They result from the metaphysical views deeply entrenched within modernity itself—metaphysical views themselves based on an instrumental approach to and subsequent alienation from the world and, consequently, from ourselves.

The metaphysics of modernity

During the twentieth century a variety of philosophers have analyzed and criticized the characteristic metaphysical structure inherent within modern culture. What we might refer to as the metaphysics of modernity, a structure of thought which, far from being specific to philosophical culture, can be seen as implicit in modern culture in general, might be brought into focus if we return to the origins of modern science. Traditionally such moves toward "objectivity" implicit in these sciences—the move from the immediate perceptually based knowledge of the cosmos to the universe of modern physics, or from the patient's own felt knowledge of their illness to the doctor's knowledge articulated in terms of the pathological functioning of physiological systems—have been interpreted as a simple transition from ignorance or error to knowledge or truth. The relation between a patient's account of their illness and the doctor's reconstruction could be seen as analogous to the difference between an everyday description of a body in terms of its color or a description of the sun moving across the sky on the one hand and a scientific description of the frequency of reflected light or a description of the dynamics of our solar system on the other. The former accounts may be adequate to the (mere) appearance of things but do not capture their underlying "reality." Just as the everyday world has to be rejected in the growth of science, so does the first-person description of an illness have to be rejected in the development of its scientific understanding.

Such an interpretation is not philosophically innocent but is underlaid by definite "metaphysical" ideas. It presupposes a definite metaphysical theory according to which the move to objectivity is seen as progress toward a knowledge of how the world is "in itself" or how it is "anyhow," independent of the ways we relate to it. Despite its apparent scientificity, such a theory, many have argued, is bound up with theological notions as deep as those buried in the medieval worldview that the modern scientific one replaced.

Indeed, in the early period of modern philosophy this goal of objective scientific knowledge was explicitly identified with *God's* knowledge of the world: science gave, literally, a "God's-eye view" of the world.[12] This was knowledge of the world to be had from some "place" where the knowing subject could be free of any actual conditions that effected the knowledge; that is, the knowledge could not be seen in any real sense as something that belonged to the world. On such a view of things, the subject who knew could therefore not be regarded in any real sense as embodied, as such embodiment, tying the knowledge to worldly conditions and perspectives, would compromise it.[13] For Descartes, then, as for many after him, the knowing subject was a very different type of thing to the body—a nonspatial, nontemporal spiritual type of substance, a "mind." To the extent that the mind was, as a matter of (perhaps regrettable) fact, linked to a body, this body played the role of a type of constrainer of knowledge, an annoying source of error.

Within modern philosophy, this debate has been played out between the supporters of the view that science ideally tells us about the world "in itself"— the "scientific realists"—and the critics of this view who see the God's-eye view conception of knowledge as an irrelevant model for human knowledge.[14] It is crucial to stress that what is at issue here are philosophical theories about science rather than questions that can be answered within the sciences themselves. The doctor, for example, will be thinking within the field of science when she answers questions about the cause of this disease or the likely physical manifestations of that one. But once the question of whether the scientific conception of disease captures something that is really there, independent of the way in which the knower is related to it (the disease "in itself" as it were), then the issue becomes a philosophical one. Consequently, the doctor who dismisses the patient's view of his or her disease as a merely erroneous view of a reality captured correctly from the scientific point of view is moving from the scientific to the philosophical terrain; she is also making a judgment which, from the point of view of those critics of realism, is deeply flawed.

An alternative philosophical interpretation of the relation of the doctor's and the patient's forms of knowledge is that each is suitable for a different practical relation of the knower to that which is known, the disease. From this point of view the concern is no longer with which account of the disease is correct in general; rather, it is with differentiating those contexts for which different types of knowledge may be relevant or irrelevant, helpful or dangerous. As we have identified the knowledge of modern science as significant within the context of an instrumental intervention into the body as a system, the question raised concerns the limits and alternatives to such a relation to the body. But as the modern sciences presuppose such a relation as the framework of knowledge, it would be circular to think that such questions could be answerable within science.

Reinstating the communication between doctors and patients: the benefits of a hermeneutic approach

In the search for alternative frameworks for reflection about medical knowledge and practice, recently some attention has been directed to the tradition of hermeneutic thought.[15] Given the nature of the perceived limitations of the natural science model—its reinterpretation of the patient from intentional and expressive subject to deterministic mechanism—the motives for such a turn can be readily understood. The discipline of hermeneutics has always been concerned with the interpretation of forms of human intentional expression and has long opposed the reduction of human existence to the mechanisms studied by natural science. Originating in techniques of textual exegesis, hermeneutics became broadened in the early twentieth century to a philosophical framework for the human sciences and attempted to demonstrate their conceptual and methodological autonomy from the forms of explanation found in the natural sciences. For Wilhelm Dilthey in particular, the idea of knowledge as the ability to predict was irrelevant for humanistic studies such as history or psychology. While the task of the natural sciences was to subsume the particular event under general deterministic causal laws, that of the human sciences was to come to an understanding of human lives in terms of the cultural frameworks of meaning within which they were experienced and lived—frameworks such as that of language in which meaning was objectified and culturally transmitted.[16]

We can now see how a manifestation of disease might be alternatively regarded. Within a naturalistic epistemology, a symptom will be interpreted as a meaningless effect of some underlying causal process. Hermeneutically, however, it will be seen as occupying a place within the complex network of meaningful relations constituting the "life-world" of the patient's experience and action.[17] A hermeneutically sensitive physician would therefore be attuned to the significance assumed by the symptoms in terms of the role they played within this life-world. Besides the skills of clinical diagnosis she would need (and so need to be trained in) the sorts of skills more commonly found in the anthropologist or the biographer. Furthermore, hermeneutic knowledge might be seen as entering into an understanding of the very goal at which a therapy aims. While from a biological point of view, "well-being" might be thought of as normal functioning, from a hermeneutic point of view such well-being could only be assessed in terms of the sort of life that the patient found subjectively meaningful and worth living. The possible outcomes of various therapies, for example, would have to be assessed against this background, not that of the "normal" functioning of a deterministic biological system.[18]

While such an increasing sensitivity to the world of the patient might be applauded, there are nevertheless limitations to the extent that Dilthey's conception of hermeneutics could be taken to provide a broader framework for reflection and judgment in clinical practice. While providing the idea of another way of thinking to challenge the tendency to "scientism" that often seems to naturally accompany an appreciation of the power of science, this classical "Diltheian" approach to hermeneutics can still be criticized as remaining captive of that invisible culture I have referred to as modern metaphysics. Dilthey simply adds a new dimension to our existence: besides being biological machines, we are also bearers of cultural formations. The scientific expertise of the doctor manipulating the disease needs to be augmented by a quite separate hermeneutic expertise in "understanding" it.

Such epistemological dualism (for which the world falls apart into two distinct realms—nature and culture—each to be studied by its distinct methodology) might itself be seen as problematic for the medical realm. Phenomena such as psychosomatic diseases and hysterical conversion reactions, together with what is known concerning the role of subjective stress in the pathogenesis and course of many organic diseases, suggest that the world turns a deaf ear to Diltheian dichotomies. The realms of nature and culture, causality and meaning, simply seem to refuse to keep their respective grounds.[19]

A more philosophically challenging and, perhaps, medically relevant hermeneutic response to the privileging of the knowledge of the natural sciences comes from the work of a contemporary German philosopher, Hans-Georg Gadamer. Gadamer has an essentially pluralistic view of knowledge: the reductive explanatory schemata of natural science are one form that human knowledge can take; the hermeneutic "understanding" of another's world is another. But Gadamer rejects the underlying metaphysical assumptions that lead us to ask which forms of knowledge get their objects "right" in any abstract sense. His refusal of the idea of a "world in itself" to be mirrored in knowledge avoids locking thought into the sharp nature/culture dichotomy characteristic of Diltheian hermeneutics.[20]

This pluralist position does not lead, as some have claimed, to an ultimate skepticism or relativism. Gadamer acknowledges science's "unassailable authority" for us; he simply suggests that we cannot in turn find any philosophical answer to the question of the rational grounds of this authority. We cannot justify our acceptance of science by the claims that it ideally gives us a comprehensive ultimate description of the world "in itself"—a God's-eye view of the world that will be the final judge of all other views. Rejecting philosophical projects which search for the certain grounds of knowledge allows him to pose different kinds of questions about science, such as his question, quoted earlier, about how we reconnect science's power "with those fundamental orders of our being that are never arbitrary or manipulable by us, but rather, simply demand respect."[21]

What Gadamer seems to be doing with the idea of such orders of our being is reminding us of our essential finitude and mortality and, by implication, of the finitude and mortality of our intellectual products, including our science. If scientific knowledge construes the world as under the power of our prediction and control, we must acknowledge as mythical the image of our ever attaining a comprehensive knowledge of the world per se. Such a myth would amount to a self-deifying image of ourselves as in a position to predict and control the world per se and would hence repress the fact that we ourselves belong essentially to that world.

In medicine, being conscious of the mythical traps of thinking of ourselves in this way might amount to acknowledging that some aspects of our lives, certain amounts of physical and psychological pain for example, are just that—aspects of life rather than contexts appropriate for the technological intervention of the "cure." The current enthusiasm in some quarters for cryogenics might be seen as symptomatic of the desire to regard death per se as a treatable illness rather than a necessary and unavoidable boundary of life.

From such a perspective we will see that it is useless to look within science for the sort of criteria that can help us in our need to integrate science into the framework of our lives. Certainly this does not mean that some other comprehensive discourse—religion, for example, or its modern dreamed of replacement of a science of ethics—can provide it, either. And if no single discourse is unilaterally authoritative, then this also excludes individual patients' own understandings of their healthy or diseased states. There is no *ultimate* authority in Gadamer's world, only a plurality of limited and defeasible authorities. Concomitantly, there can be no overarching authoritative univocal discourse within which the competing claims of different human discourses can be measured and definitively assessed. He is able to avoid the relativistic implications of the mere fragmentation of authority, however, by providing a model for a wider context within which we should view such univocal discourses as interaction: this is the model of dialogue.

Within a dialogue each partner speaks for a position that cannot be collapsed into the other. Such an event would reduce it to a collective monologue: the voice of a unified "we" in which the separation of the reciprocal roles of "I" and "you" was lost. As such, the dialogue provides a model of a communicative event in which separate horizons of intelligibility interact but never completely merge in an act of one subsuming the other.[22]

We might see the Gadamerian dialogue as providing a model for thinking about the communicative interaction between patient and doctor in a way that avoids the idea that the scientific perspective of the latter reductively subsumes the experiential, lived perspective of the former. Rather, each speaking position interprets one dimension of the shared object of concern—the disease—at the cost of obscuring another: the doctor discloses the disease as a thing manipulable from the outside; the patient sees it as a thing lived with from the inside.

From such a point of view the doctor's understanding of the disease from the horizon of science must always remain open to the claims made from that of the life-world of the patient. In other words, the doctor must appreciate that, within the patient's discourse, real claims are being made about something that escapes capture from the scientific perspective; furthermore, claims have their own type of truth that must be taken seriously into account in the course of dealing with the disease. In many respects the same thing must also be done by the patient. The "fact" of the disease is not something totally knowable from any single point of view. There is always a side to the body and its states which escapes the concepts brought from either lived "first-person" or scientific "third-person" accounts. The sick body is something that exists within an open-ended and dialogical therapeutic interaction in which neither point of view can claim ultimate authority.

Acknowledging the voice of the patient

The limits of the univocal technoscientific interpretation of the medical domain are perhaps most apparent in those contexts where doctors are faced with patients suffering from illnesses for which there simply are no existing cures. In such situations, the underlying conception of an illness as a dysfunctional state for intervention and rectification suggest the interpretation that "Here there is nothing that can be done." And yet diseases that cannot be cured must be lived or died with, and in this matter the doctor's knowledge and attention is no less relevant: it simply needs to be engaged in a different way. Now the goal of the interaction becomes that of integrating the brute, objective understanding of the disease borne by the doctor into the lived perspective of the patient, and this goal *explicitly* demands a dialogical interaction between the two and their different perspectives. Not only will this integration be crucial for the patient's management of his or her own life with the disease but also it is essential for the mitigation of that aspect of suffering which accompanies the feeling of the *meaninglessness* of one's own pain.

Giving pain an interpretation may not cure it, but it can help counter some of the fragmenting effects pain can have on a person's life.[23] While the value of "communicating" with the patient is often stressed in the medical context, the instrumental model can even tend to construe this as something done by the doctor *to* the patient: "information" and advice being dispensed like drugs with the assumption that they can be causally effective in something like the same way. From a Gadamerian framework, knowledge cannot be conveyed like a thing to a passive recipient. It is only as a response to the questioning arising from the own lived perspective that communicated knowledge can become integrated into the world of the patient.

To see knowledge as part of the fabric of the world as Gadamer does, rather than something standing over against it and reflecting it, means that questions of knowledge can only artificially be kept separate from those of its worldly distribution and control. Accordingly, Gadamer's view of science draws our attention to the ethical and political dimensions of questions of knowledge.

As a number of commentators have suggested, the view of science advocated in the wake of the successes of modern physics in the early modern period was far from being free of religious and political connotations. Descartes and Galileo linked the authority of physics to religion by conceiving of God as a mathematician.[24] Similarly, later in the seventeenth century Newton saw himself as working out the structure of those general laws governing the universe which had themselves been decreed by a transcendent God. He saw his physics as intimately connected with both theology and politics because in all realms order was properly established in a homologous way, that is, hierarchically from above down.[25]

Probably there is no clearer case of such a linking of political authority with the authority of science than that of the modern doctor. As long as doctors have been able to draw on the conception of science as *the* authority about the world, they have been able to legitimize a claim to always "know what is best" for their patients. The equation of the subjective view based on experience with simple error, to be corrected by scientific truth, has helped keep patients disenfranchised in the governance of their own corporeal selves. Acknowledging that the voice of the patient carries its own distinctive authority means challenging the accepted distribution of power and authority within the institutions of medicine. If questions of the nature of medical knowledge cannot be untangled from those of medical ethics, neither can they be untangled from questions of medical politics.

Notes

1   The work of historian of science, Thomas Kuhn, has been crucial here. See his *Copernican Revolution* (Cambridge, Mass., Harvard University Press, 1957) and *The Structure of Scientific Revolutions* (Chicago, University of Chicago Press, 1962).

2 Cf. Hans Blumenberg, *The Genesis of the Copernican World*, trans. Robert M. Wallace (Cambridge, Mass., MIT Press, 1987).

3 This theme is developed by Karsten Harries in "Copernican Reflections and the Tasks of Metaphysics," *International Philosophical Quarterly* 23 (1983): 235–252, and in "Copernican Reflections," *Inquiry* 23 (1980): 252–269.

4 Cf. Rene Descartes, *Principles of Philosophy*, in *The Philosophical Writings of Descartes*, trans. J. Cottingham, R. Stoothoff, and D. Murdoch (Cambridge: Cambridge University Press, 1985), vol. 1, pp. 217–218; and Galileo, "The Assayer," reprinted in A. Danto and S. Morgengesser, eds., *Philosophy of Science* (Cleveland, Meridian Books, 1960), p. 28.

5 Claude Bernard, *Introduction à l'etude de la medicine expérimentale* (Paris, J. B Baillièrs, 1865), trans. H. C. Grene as *An Introduction to the Study of Experimental Medicine*, (New York, Macmillan, 1927). The work of French epistemologist Georges Canguilhem has been crucial in demonstrating the "epistemological rupture" initiated by Bernard's concept of internal environment. See his *The Normal and the Pathological*, trans. C. R. Fawcett and Robert S. Cohen (Dordrecht, D. Reidel, 1978). The idea of an epistemological rupture, which comes from the work of Gaston Bachelard, parallels Thomas Kuhn's notion of "paradigm shift" in signaling the radical discontinuities in knowledge involved in the growth of the sciences.

6 For a general discussion of the history of these issues, see Stephen Toulmin, *Cosmopolis* (Chicago, University of Chicago Press, 1990).

7 For example, by Max Horkheimer and Theodor Adorno in *The Dialectic of Enlightenment*, trans. J. Cumming (London, Allen Lane, 1973).

8 H.-G. Gadamer, *Philosophical Hermeneutics*, transl. David E. Linge (Berkeley, University of California Press, 1976), p. 3.

9 Ibid., pp. 3–4.

10 See, for example, Alasdair Macintyre, *After Virtue* (Duckworth, London, 1981) and Bernard Williams, *Ethics and the Limits of Philosophy* (London, Fontana paperback, 1985). For the relevance of this type of critique of moral philosophy to bioethics, see Max Charlesworth, "Bioethics and the Limits of Philosophy," *Bioethics News* 9 no. 1 (Oct. 1989), pp. 9–25.

11 The approach of Martin Heidegger has been crucial here.

12 A clear account of the theological dimensions of early modern epistemology can be found in Edward Craig, *The Mind of God and the Works of Man* (Oxford, Clarendon Press, 1987).

13 Cf., Karsten Harries, "Descartes, Perspective and the Angelic Eye," *Yale French Studies*, 49 (1973): 28–42.

14 For an overview, see, for example, Richard J. Bernstein, *Beyond Objectivism and Relativism* (Oxford, Blackwell, 1983).

15 See, for example, a recent issue of the journal *Theoretical Medicine* (Vol. 11, no. 1, March 1990) devoted to the topic of medical hermeneutics. Besides the special issue, this journal has regularly published contributions on this topic, as has the *Journal of Medicine and Philosophy*.

16 Cf. Wilhelm Dilthey, *Selected Writings*, transl. and ed. H. P. Rickman (Cambridge, Cambridge University Press, 1976).

17 For an illuminating discussion of disease from the perspective of the lived-body, see Drew Leder, "Medicine and the Paradigms of Embodiment," *Journal of Medicine and Philosophy* 9 (1984): 29–43 and *The Absent Body* (Chicago, University of Chicago Press, 1990).

18   In a discussion on the ancient concept of morality as the "health of the soul," Nietzsche wrote: "There is no health as such, and all attempts to define a thing that way have been wretched failures. Even the determination of what is healthy for your *body* depends on your goal, your horizon, your energies, your impulses, your errors, and above all on the ideas and phantasms of your soul." Friedrich Nietzsche, *The Gay Science,* transl. Walter Kaufmann (New York, Vintage Books, 1974 (first published in German in 1882)), pp. 176–77.

19   It has been argued that, under the impetus of recent research linking psychology, immunology, endocrinology, and neurology, "it is reasonable to expect that there will be an increasing *convergence* between *the body of medicine and the body of lived experience*" (David Michael Levin and George F. Solomon, "The Discursive Formation of the Body," *Journal of Medicine and Philosophy* 15 [1990]: p. 533). These issues are complex and require much clarification at a conceptual level. From what I have argued about the instrumentalist construction of the "body of medicine," it is difficult to see how "convergence" here is to be understood. The difficulty and ambiguity of issues concerning the relation between hermeneutic and scientific approaches to the body, together with the question of the degree to which science is itself a form of hermeneutic interpretation, is reflected in some of the conflicts in the literature. See for example the differences between Drew Leder, "Clinical Interpretation: The Hermeneutics of Medicine," and Richard J. Baron, "Medical Hermeneutics: Where Is the Text We Are Interpreting?" both in *Theoretical Medicine,* Vol. 11 no. 1, (1990), as well as the critique of Leder's article by Larry R. Churchill, "Hermeneutic in Science and Medicine: A Thesis Understated," in the following issue.

20   Gadamer's magnum opus (first published in German in 1960) is *Truth and Method,* transl. William Glen-Doepel (London, Sheed and Ward, 1975). A more accessible introduction to his thought is via the essays in *Reason in the Age of Science,* transl. Frederick G. Lawrence (Cambridge, Mass., MIT Press, 1981).

21   See note 9. For an excellent discussion of Gadamer's interpretation of science, see Michael Kelly, "On Hermeneutics and Science: Why Hermeneutics Is Not Anti-science," *Southern Journal of Philosophy* 25 (1987): 481–500.

22   See Gadamer, *Truth and Method,* pp. 320–51.

23   See Leder's discussion of pain from a phenomenological perspective in *Absent Body,* chap. 3.

24   See Craig, *Mind of God and The Works of Man,* Ch 1.

25   On Newton's extra-scientific views, see J. E. Force and R. H. Popkin, *Essays on the Context, Nature and Influence of Isaac Newton's Theology* (Kluwer, Dordrecht, 1990).

The body politic

Peter Murphy

Human beings are cultural beings. Their practices and activities are structured culturally. This is as true of the practices and activities of the body as it is of any other dimension of the *vita activa*. The sum of cultural knowledge can be expressed, precisely, in ideal types of the body. Each ideal type tells us how the body is to behave, and how it is to be treated, in a particular human culture. Each culture is composed of both norms (ethics) and values (goods), which orientate practices and activities, respectively. I do not want to suggest that cultural orientation (the orientation to norms and values) is the only aspect of the human condition. But it is a central one; one which, today, given the increasingly polyglot, or pluralized, character of human experience, stands out in the philosophical-anthropological spotlight.

Human beings, as the very condition of their humanness, live in cultural contexts.[1] For the individual in the first place this means, at one level, observance of, and orientation to, a more or less coherent, more or less given, set of forms and values. At least in some cases, however, the individual may also inhabit legal and administrative (state) structures that are shared with others whose cultural orientations are quite different. These individuals, together, will inhabit a multicultural state. Although, today, "multiculturalism" is a conspicuously vogue word, associated with sometimes dubious political lobbies, the existence and distinctive problems of multicultural states (or polyvalent societies) more or less coincide with the birth of the Western world, and are very much bound up with its fate.

Just as the Greek city-states managed for a time to find a bridge between the old Homeric warrior culture and the civic culture of an urban aristocracy, Imperial Rome shared its center with the Christians and its margins with those it colonized. Likewise, the medieval world, although nominally Christian, was, in practice, split between warrior, courtly, and churchly cultures. Of course, neither Rome nor Christendom in particular conceived of itself as just one culture among many. In their self-conception, they were of universal significance. But both the Romans and the Christians had a degree of self-consciousness about the problems of reconciling their universalistic ambitions with the specificities of the cultures they ruled over. Roman jurists, for example, took the view that all people who are governed by law and by custom observe laws that are in part their own and in part are common to all humankind. The Romans distinguished between civil law (what they called *ius civile*), which expresses the interests of one particular community; the law of nations (*ius gentium*), which facilitates mutual intercourse between communities; and the law of nature (*ius naturale*), which is observed by all humankind. The medieval Christians, especially under the influence of the revival in learning in the twelfth century, could make similar distinctions. For my purposes here, this history is significant only as a reminder of the past of our present. Our present—the present of modern Western states at least—is multicultural, as is our past. And it is both a present and a past that is, for the very fact of being multicultural, fraught with difficulty: the difficulty of reconciling antinomical cultures, of finding a basis for their civil coexistence.

To what extent, and in what way, is the civil coexistence of antinomical cultures possible? The Roman and Christian answer—a universal law that is shared by different particular cultures—came unstuck, as all subsequent universals have, because of the tendency of *ius naturale* to resemble the culture of Rome or Christendom. The universal that was supposed to be common to the denizens of all particular cultures or communities was itself a particular culture. Are then all universals merely particulars in disguise, particulars that have overreached themselves and have thereby become oppressive? Or is it, perhaps, the case that universals are not ipso facto oppressive, but they can become so, and they become so because of the failure of politics? Politics arises only in the midst of antinomical cultures. It establishes, in the words of the Roman jurists, mutual intercourse between communities. Thus, politics is closer in spirit to *ius gentium* than to either *ius naturale* or *ius civile*. In a manner of speaking, politics is the middle term between the universal and the particular. The political actor balances, diplomatically, judiciously, the claims of all communities (cultures, traditions) in the attempt to establish an equilibrium between them. But such an outcome is only ever possible, or conceivable, where cultures, notwithstanding their antinomies, share something minimal in common (an *ius naturale*) that permits them to recognize and respect each other and talk to each other and deal with each other in a civil manner. The judicious and diplomatic art of politics is all for nought if there is no fulcrum (at least one common norm or value) on which otherwise competing cultures may be balanced. The art of the political actor, who pursues the *ius gentium,* is never an easy one, and the effort to establish a political equilibrium in a multicultural state is never a simple matter, for it means that individuals have to come to terms with living in a multidimensional universe in which their cultural world, which represents everything precious and valuable to them, is brought into coexistence with other worlds that represent things indifferent or even antithetical to their own disposition. Let us turn to the case of the body to illustrate this.

Competing conceptions of the body

Within the arterial systems of contemporary Western states there circulates a number of competing conceptions of the body.

Communitarian

The first of these is the communitarian conception, which is a protective attitude. The communitarian values life, and the ethic that follows from this is one of maintaining and defending human life and of reducing threats to life and the life-world. The communitarian attitude is to some extent a secularized version of older religious attitudes, particularly but not exclusively pre-Reformation Christian, although some, especially conservative, communitarians still maintain explicit religious beliefs. The religious sense of the sacred represents one version of the communitarian ethos. Historically, however, human beings have created many different kinds of metaphors and forms for sheltering the body, not only religious ones. Among the oldest are patriarchal and patrimonial conceptions of a household order that provides, ideally, care and protection for its members in return for the obedience of those members to the household head. Of more recent, though still pre-modern, and largely European, origin is the class model of protection. In this model, membership of a social class (rather than the kinship of a household) offers the promise of solidarity against harm and injury. Added to this is the protection that upper (e.g., warrior, landlord) classes can offer vulnerable and weak status groups. In the European setting, the feudal contract was one of protection exchanged for service. And in all sorts of nominally more modern settings (e.g., turn-of-the-century American immigrant communities) political and social notables have continued to offer protection to weak or vulnerable individuals in exchange for favors.

Today, the protective significance of the household and of class has waned for human beings. Conservatives, of the right and left, will still offer the prospect of familial-household or class canopies erected as defenses against the jeopardies of modern life. But such claims have become increasingly unconvincing, partly because the hierarchical assumptions of these models cannot be sustained in an age of democratic equality, and partly because what constitutes threats to life in the modern world (e.g., uncontrolled urbanization, industrialization) takes on an increasingly depersonalized character where it is no longer powerful individuals but rather forms of social regulation that are key to reducing risks to life. This does not imply the disappearance of communitarian attitudes, but it does mean their transformation. They take on new forms. In some cases, it has meant the appearance of new kinds of household (e.g., the feminized, single-parent household); in other cases, the substitution of institutional forms of protection (e.g., job security) for patrimonial or class forms. The most spectacular example of institutional protection has been the emergence of the welfare state which provides a "safety net" in the form of state regulation of "unsafe" industrial or social practices and the provision of general or universal social insurance (health benefits, illness benefits, and so on).

The rationale of the welfare state is a "protected society." The very notion of "society" as a key locus of meaning for individuals, we should remember, is of quite recent origin. It emerged from the cauldron of the French Revolution and quickly thereafter established considerable sway over thought and politics.[2] The welfare state gradually took shape under the auspices of the idea of society. What was crucial was the notion that not just individuals but something called "society" needed to be protected—against the ravages of industrialism, capitalism, international competition, migratory waves, and so on. Whereas, in the seventeenth and eighteenth centuries in Europe, there had been considerable discussion of the way in which individuals were threatened by the predatory behavior of governments or else by other individuals who were unscrupulous or unreliable in their dealings, many in the nineteenth century began to talk as if an entity called "society" also needed to be protected from harm.

Harm to society was not understood in individualistic terms, but in terms of the "rates of incidence" of certain malign phenomena (e.g., disease, hunger, and suicide) that were found to occur within different groups that composed "society." These different groups could be compared (e.g., workers and managers, Catholics and Protestants, men and women, English and Irish, northerners and southerners), and "social problems" could be identified where higher rates of mortality or disease existed in one group as compared with another group or compared with the "social average." Such "rates of incidence" were quantifiable; they could be measured statistically (hence the emergence of the professional statistician and demographer). So could the "social causes" of "social problems." The "causes" of disease and death were traced not just to the individual organism, or psyche, but to social environments—to the (again measurable) overcrowding in cities, pollution of rivers and air, and prevalence of filthy and unsanitary conditions. In some cases, though, the "causes" of disease and death were also traced to specific social groups. In particular, various migratory, ethnic, and indigenous groups were singled out. These groups were represented, in a reversal of the normal pattern, not as suffering from a certain incidence of some "social scourge" (e.g., cholera or malnutrition), but rather as the (stated or implied, actual or potential) "cause" of a high incidence of that scourge among other groups in "society." This was, in a word, racism, and the propensity of many "socialists" and "social reformer," among others, in the nineteenth and twentieth centuries to be drawn to racist or chauvinistic beliefs and policies should not be forgotten. Nor should it be assumed that this is no longer the case. While some chauvinisms are thoroughly discredited (e.g., the kind that led to Australia's anti-Chinese "White Australia" policy), others flourish, often under fashionable banners like "postcolonialism" (ironically enough) or "social ecology." They avoid the discredit of earlier chauvinisms by recasting (sometimes simply by inverting) those who, in their moral play, are the "harmful groups" (e.g., North American WASP consumers) and those who are the groups "at risk." But the "good group"/"bad group" thinking—vaguely reminiscent of some archaic communalism—remains unchanged, and today, as in the past, it is often tacitly legitimated by the probabilistic social sciences, whose own assumptions, especially in the hands of reductive practitioners, lend themselves all too easily to this abuse. Neither the "social" sciences nor "social" movements can claim immunity from the temptation to descent into the cesspool of biopolitics. Indeed, this is their peculiar weakness.

The link between "social" science and "social" prescription was, from the beginning, a close one. The statistician—or else that other offspring of the nineteenth century, the sociologist—could identify which groups were subject to what kind of environment, and could form correlations between environment, group, and the frequency of death or disease. "Social reformers"—many of them self-described socialists or social liberals—then offered prescriptions, mainly in the form of social regulations, for breaking the nexus between social "problem" and "cause." Regulation by public health and other authorities offered the promise of reducing overcrowding, ensuring the hygienic handling of foodstuffs, guaranteeing adequate air and light in houses, and so forth. Over time, this "social protection" model was extended to the workplace (regulation of factories to reduce the incidence of injury and debilitation among workers) and to the marketplace (regulation of rates of pay to establish a "living wage"). While such examples of regulation were not in themselves unprecedented—we need only think, for example, of the building regulations adopted after the Great Fire of London in 1666—what was unprecedented was the allying of regulation to the concept of "society." The administration of public health, occupational safety, and so forth, was preventive, and what it prevented (in theory, at least) were the environmental conditions that "caused" social problems, and this was done in order to "protect society," which amounted to reducing the incidence of the spread of disease, death, and injury among statistically recognized groups in "society."

This is far removed from the solidaristic ethos, or *caritas*, of earlier forms of communitarianism. Such earlier forms stimulated feelings that the world was a dependable place—a solid place—because there were at least some people in the world, people known and encountered in everyday life, who were "loyal" and "good," who could assist, or if not that, at least console, those who were exposed to the hazards of life. The modern welfare state exhibits little of the face-to-face emotional contact typical of earlier communitarian forms. Yet it manages to inspire both great reforming (evangelical) enthusiasm on the part of "social reformers" and feelings of security on the part of beneficiaries of modern welfare; in so doing, it manages to simulate an ersatz sense of community. Indeed, the need to "feel secure" has become a central preoccupation in late modern societies. This is, at least partly, because of the complexity of these societies, and the resulting ambivalences and uncertainties they generate. It is also, partly, simply what these societies are, and one of the consequences of this has been the development, in the twentieth century, of fiscal alongside regulatory welfare, with the state providing benefits in the case that individuals get ill or injured, or are exposed to the prospect of destitution and its potentially debilitating impact. Unlike regulatory welfare, fiscal welfare does not aim at removing the "causes" of "social problems," but it does, all the same, follow the logic of regulatory welfare in maintaining that individuals are not (ever) the responsible causes of injury, illness, or death (whether their own or somebody else's). In this conception, it is the factory system, not the negligent manager, that is responsible for causing the injury; the hazards of the modern highway system, not the incompetent driver, are at fault.

The effect of the fiscal welfarism has been double-edged. It unquestionably gives the denizens of late modern societies the feelings of security that they crave. And yet it does not give them any feelings of confidence in the world and in their capacities to act in the world. Because the "social environment," as the welfare state mentality conceives of it, is constantly interpreted as malign or threatening, it does not give people confidence to go out into the world and act with a sense of purpose and initiative. The world, in other words, is a "bad" place. People may "know" (and "feel secure" in the knowledge) that they "are covered" if catastrophe strikes (they have hospital insurance, sickness benefits, etc.). But, at the same time, they "know" they are not the "cause" of what happens in the world. They are not effective agents, and to assume otherwise would mean to undermine the presuppositions of the welfare state paradigm. Nor can they even influence those who are effective agents, because (in contemporary parlance) it is systems (factories, markets, offices, etc.) that "act," not agents. The "cost" of this is not only the loss of confidence by agents in their capacities to act but also a lack of a sense of responsibility for action ("It wasn't me who caused the injury, it was the faulty system, the lousy procedure"), a state of affairs which, ironically, mimics (or is it parodies?)—at least in consequence—the "childishness" of those subject to the care and protection of the old patrimonial and pastoral orders, with one added vice, that this state of affairs is offered as a model for all classes and groups in "society."

Rational ascetic

The rational ascetic attitude toward the body is methodical. As has often been observed, in Western states, rational ascetic attitudes had a monastic origin, but became of more generalized cultural significance in the early modern period. The aim of rational asceticism is to subject the body to a systematic regime of rational conduct (where the terms systematic and rational are more or less synonymous). Rational asceticism "disciplines" the body. Its expectation is that the body will behave (or move) in methodical and regular ways. This has, above all, an "economic" significance. Rational asceticism eradicates whatever is impulsive or spontaneous ("irrational"), and thus unpurposeful or undirected, in bodily actions. Rational asceticism emphasizes the virtues of conscientiousness—virtues that are expressed in the careful and methodical way a person pursues a task, problem, issue, or calling. The regime of conscientious virtue both prohibits actions (e.g., wasting time, idleness) and institutes methodical practices. But its significance lies not just in its normative constraint or "discipline"; it also creates a kind of freedom. This is not, of course, the communitarian kind—the promise of freedom from life-threatening hazards. It is a freedom that arises from the fact that rational asceticism encourages individuals to make deliberate choices about their bodies. Methodicality implies greater deliberateness (forethought, calculation, etc.) in human behavior, and that deliberateness puts human beings in a situation where they have to make (yes/no) choices about how they are going to act.

Rational ascetic attitudes shape not only the actions but also the understanding, and the treatment, of the body, as we can see from the case of modern medicine. Modern medicine is driven by scientific discovery. It advances with corresponding advances in medical research—research that is, like all modern science, deeply indebted to and inconceivable without rational asceticism. Modern (empirical-analytic) science defines itself methodologically. The doing of "scientific" research is painstakingly methodical. This methodicality involves the analytic dissection or division of a problem domain into its parts (into cases, incidences, and examples), along with the systematic examination of these parts—their precise observation, accurate recording, structured comparison, and so on.

Ideally, the observer acts "coolly," "dispassionately," "logically"—taking note of how each specimen, each example, each test subject behaves; doing this in terms of the analytically distinct elements that, for analytical-empirical science, make up each observable object; describing regularities and variations, consistencies and inconsistencies, standard results and anomalies—doing so, time, after time, after time, to "see" whether the data (the meticulous, careful recording of observations) confirms some hypothesis or some speculation of the researcher. In this speculation, the researcher anticipates some regularity—for example, in the course of the development of a disease—some causal sequence that orders events in nature. Such speculation is nothing, however, without the confirmation of observation. And just as the "discipline" of empirical-analytic science demands that the "hunches" of the researcher be confirmed by observational data, it also demands that the observations of individual researchers are consistent with, or at least in some significant way converge, or overlap, with the observations of other researchers. Here again precision is crucial—precision, this time, in language usage, in the ways in which what is observed is designated, otherwise what is recorded will be incommensurable with the data of other researchers and useless for purposes of confirmation or refutation. As is the case in all "disciplines," there are, of course, in practice, those who are better or worse attuned to the "discipline" of empirical-analytical science, for reasons of either aptitude or principle. There is also always, alas, the intractable opacity of language, its native resistance to the analytic drive for pure transparency, and its coloring by the theoretical and programmatic assumptions that tacitly shape any observational language and ignite ambivalences where the analyst demands clarity.

Much, therefore, ultimately eludes the aspiration of empirical-analytic science for transparency and regularity. Yet it is this aspiration that nonetheless shapes, fundamentally, what this science is and what it does. Notwithstanding the role played by creative insight and good intuitions (postrational hypothesizing and speculating), the culture of modern research science is one of rigor, not one of spontaneity, and this conditions what medical science can and cannot know, and what modern medicine is and is not. When the body becomes the object of science, it becomes the object of systematic, analytical examination. This is so whether we are talking of research or of medical consultation and hospital practice. The 15-minute consultation, with its clinical examination and precise exchange between doctor and patient about symptoms, and its exclusion, more or less, of any comforting, consoling, or commiserating with the patient; the strictures of hospital routine; the departmentalization and bureaucratization of health care, and so on—all have their origins in the culture of rational asceticism, and all share the strengths and weaknesses of that culture. What that culture does well is to encourage deliberateness in human affairs. It encourages people to look at the relationships between causes and effects, between means and ends, and to break up problematic wholes into parts that can be systematically and sequentially worked through. It encourages people to deal with the world in "rational" ways—i.e., not affective, or mystical, or stoical,—but which involve the deliberate establishment of a step-by-step course of action (a course of treatment, a research program, etc.). The most positive consequence of such methodical deliberateness is that it can free people from the arbitrary and mysterious forces of superstition, fate, magic, happenstance, and fortune. This empowerment, and this freedom, however, can turn back and devour itself, so that methods become hypertrophied, plans inflexible, organization routine, and choices impersonal, and gradually an apparatus replaces individual calculation and deliberation.

Much of the criticism of the practice of modern medicine is, in effect, a criticism of its failure to fulfill its promise of rationality. It is a criticism of the way in which rational ascetic "rationality" that gave modern medicine its identity and distinctive attitude to the body frequently lapses into the pseudorationality of bureaucracy. It is quite obvious that for many, indeed most, of those who enter the "medical system," whether as patients, nurses, paramedical professionals, or even doctors, the institutionalization of that system—which the culture of rational asceticism and its preference for methodical organization encourages—insistently confounds individual deliberateness, and, in effect, leads to the reestablishment of a regime of "arbitrary and mysterious" forces—this time, organizational ones. One of the ironies of the critique of the bureaucratization of the treatment of the body is that, for all the sound and fury it can generate, it is immanent—that is, it supposes the ideal of what it criticizes. It wants to restore the promise of empowerment that rational asceticism originally offered. This contrasts, quite sharply, with the critique that comes from the communitarian quarter.

The communitarian is much less concerned with rationality. From the communitarian viewpoint, modern medicine is deficient because it neglects the pre-rational aspects of the whole person e.g., their fears, anxieties, and despair in the face of their own mortality or grief and sorrow in the face of the loss of others. Because the medical doctor treats the body "scientifically," so the communitarian argues, the "feeling" aspect of the body is bracketed. This, of course, is an overstatement. While it is true to say that there are certain types of feelings that rational asceticism tends to exclude—affections (sexual affects, fear, anxiety, shame, gaiety, sadness, tension, relief) that are bound up with our sense of (social or physical) preservation—rational asceticism, emphasizes cognitive orientational feelings (yes/no feelings) that guide us through complex situations or have a role in solving problems: feelings of probability, doubt, certainty, expectancy, and curiosity.[3] In other words, what the "medical model" cannot deal with are the pre-rational or noncognitive feelings. The often-times paralyzing and debilitating fears that people have cannot be treated medically because they demand the very communion with others (through affectionate embracing and reassurance, ritualized communal affirmations, acts of solidarity that cultivate feelings of belonging, and consensual modes of interaction and decision making) that constitutes, from a rational ascetic point of view, an "uneconomic" and "unsystematic" distraction, and thus a vice. For this reason, such communitarian neologisms as "community medicine" (progressive version) or "family medicine" (conservative version) are nothing more than fantasies. The institution of modern medicine, like the rational ascetic culture it derives from, is a cold one. It relies on analytic detachment. For all those many ailments or diseases of the body that admit of "systematic" or "methodological" treatment, however, this very coldness is not at all a vice, but a virtue.

Republican

The third attitude toward the body is the republican. The republican attitude has both a stoic and an epicurean dimension. The republican, in the first place, evinces a stoic attitude to the body. Insofar as the body is the site of affects (fear, grief, anguish, and sorrow) the stoic attitude is to bear those feelings without being overwhelmed by them. Republican personalities react with fortitude and dignity to the cruelties and pain, misfortunes and injuries, visited upon the body. For the stoic, impassiveness in the face of the threats of disease or death means not attempting to control things that are effectively beyond the control of individuals. Fearfulness, grief, etc., arise when the very things human beings value (e.g., our life, the life of another) are threatened by forces that we cannot dictate. Ironically, such pre-rational feelings paralyze us—or, as in the case of hope, put us in the unhelpful position of waiting for the arrival of a savior to extricate us from our predicament—and, in doing so, compound our lack of control, making of us undignified and cowed beings or else beings who "lash out" in anger, wildly and indiscriminately out of control, helpless and powerless. The stoical virtues—of restraint, temperance, fortitude, and courage—are meant to break this vicious cycle. And they can do so, because one thing at least—the observance of the (stoical) virtues—is always within our control, and when and where we do observe these virtues, we can resist being caught up in overwhelming and crushing pre-rational feelings of panic and urgency. It is always possible for the tired, the exhausted, the oppressed, the disease-racked to assert in the face of their suffering a kind of human autonomy—a moral autonomy—which is at the same time a kind of independence or freedom. In doing so, they can break the domination of those pre-rational affects that can very easily subsume a human life.

To be dominated by feelings of fear, grief, or panic is to be paralyzed in action, and for the republican, of course, action (public deeds) is the highest value. The sensitivity of republican personalities to the question of pre-rational feelings stems, in significant measure, from the fact that public action invariably has attendant risks, whether these are figurative or actual. There is always an element of agonal contest in public life. In civil societies, the risk is purely figurative, yet even in these societies, persons typically remain reluctant (fearful) to stand up in public—and, in Hannah Arendt's terms, distinguish themselves[4]—for fear of being annihilated. The communitarian attitude to such risks is to find protective shelters from the agonistics of public life (in the name of fostering "cooperation"). The republican attitude is to simply live with the risks of agonistics, understanding that they are an inevitable part of the life of citizens or public actors, and that public actors cannot afford to be cowed by them. Republican personalities, unsurprisingly, therefore, emphasize and rely on the virtue of courage—not the courage, incidentally, of the warrior, but the kind of civic courage needed to cope with the conflicts, tensions, and confrontations of a public world. The republican self does not look for reassurance as the communitarian does, or to the "warm" protective embrace of a community. But this does not mean that the republican lacks, as often does the rational ascetic personality, the human interest in involvement with others. What the republican personality is disinterested in is a pre-rational communion with others. For the republican personality, the key involvement with others is friendship and friendship-style loves and relationships. This is the epicurean dimension of republicanism. Friendship is quite unlike the undifferentiated mass of a community. It involves choice (selection). The feelings of friendship are what Agnes Heller describes as orientational feelings.[5] They have a crucial rational or cognitive (yes/no) dimension, and thus, for the epicurean, circles of friendship—constituted as "little republics"—are quite unlike the fraternal and claustrophobic togetherness that binds the community-minded into their *Gemeinschaft*-like shelters of mutual protection. Circles of friendship are, rather, based on elective affinity. Friends are drawn to each other because of who they are, and because of what each does and values, not because of a need to find some kind of mutual protection against real or imagined jeopardies in the world. Friends do not hold onto each other for reassurance. They embrace because each one of them is the embodiment of something valuable, attractive, and precious for the other one. The look, the gesture, the touch of each is a reminder for the other that there is value and enjoyment, as well as malignity and morbidity, in the world, and this reminder, this recollection, is a stimulus and replenisher of the confidence of each, in turn, to go out, embrace the world, and be an actor in it.

Humanistic
The fourth attitude toward the body is the humanistic. The humanistic attitude is preoccupied with the appearances of the body.[6] The humanist body is a site of display. Societies and groups (different cultures) offer their denizens particular ways of appearing to others: clothing, adornment, cosmetics, masks, etc., for the body; gymnastic and calisthenic cultivation of the body; typical kinds of gesture and body language; the forms of dance, mime, theatrical presentation; various kinds of ascetic discipline; and elocutionary or oratorical training of

the voice. These constitute forms of expression or representation for the body as it enters the public spaces of appearance where it is seen, heard, and remembered by others.

On one level, humanism can simply be a curiosity about different forms of appearance that are to be found in different cultures or different setting, in that the humanist attitude to the body is one of concern with its multiple or variegated appearances. The humanist is not distinguished by preservatory concerns, or by analytic or agonistic ones, but by the concern with exploring the richness and diversity of human appearances. The humanist is the first properly multicultural figure, inasmuch as the humanist collects the forms of appearance (masks, costumes, perfumes, etc.) from across the spectrum of human cultures and groups, and works at understanding them, at deciphering their meaning, locating them in context of the "objective mind" (Dilthey) of society or culture, and at translating between cultures. The humanist values learning, and teaching, about different forms of the body. Central to humanism is the virtue of tolerance. The antithesis of the humanist attitude is puritanical narrowness and dogmatism. The presence of humanism always has a fertilizing and broadening effect. It introduces, or reintroduces, to the world—through education and learning—"alien," "exotic," "archaic," "lost," "forgotten," "classical" traditions of regard for the body. Yet, in doing this, its interest or animating purpose is never evangelical. It doesn't have "persuasion" as its objective. It is, in fact, deeply skeptical of idealizing ardour—of intolerant, narrow, and more often than not simply ignorant evangelical and puritanical posturing—that seeks to proselytize one way of appearing, one strict demeanor, one "right" and "wrong" way of dressing and embellishing the body.

Usually the puritan opts for "plainness" in appearance. What this often means, in practice, is that the puritanically minded despises or hates appearances per se. This is because appearances are felt to distract from something "higher," "more essential," "more serious." By contrast, the humanist, in defending the plurality of appearances, often has to defend the value of appearances per se, and, in doing so, has to answer the question of what value is it that appearances have, and, in particular, what value do the appearances of the body have? Partly, the answer to this question is simply that the sheer order to enter the public spaces of appearance—constitutes an incalculable human treasure or richness. But diversity, alone, is not sufficient to explain the value of appearances. Appearances—in general, and of the body in particular—please and displease. Variety is one reason why appearances please, but not the only, nor even the principal, reason. Human beings also look to the shape, or form, in which things and bodies are presented, and variety, without shape or form, is displeasing. Just as the display of the person who collects a large number of busts, items of jewelry, or figurative paintings from different places and periods, without a thought to the overall coherence or pattern of the collection, will fail to please, so will the person who likes polychromatic attire but has no sense of what colors go together and what colors clash. Some sense of proportion or balance—be it in the presentation of bodies or in the way such presentations are housed and preserved by collectors, museums, educators, and publishers—is as important for the humanist as the sheer variety of appearances. A "lack of balance" in the way the body is presented is as likely to provoke the ire of the humanist as the monotony that results from either provincial narrowness or from puritanical zealotry.

In the modern age, the "love of appearances" is often the source of great controversy. Both the communitarian and the rational ascetic (although for different reasons) are deeply suspicious of the humanist's valuing of appearances. For the communitarian, it is unnecessary; for the rational ascetic, it is a distraction. For both it detracts from the "real business" of life. Neither the communitarian nor the rational ascetic can, for example, make much sense of the contemporary interest in cosmetic surgery. Of course, a lot of hypocrisy surrounds such a subject. When individuals, whoever they are, are confronted with the extremes of deformity, they will generally turn away from the sight (or else hide it from sight), so there is, in practice, little ethical argument about the surgical correction of gross deformity when it can be done. Yet, at the same time, the moral hounds will bay at the mention of elective cosmetic surgery—or indeed any cosmetic procedure or application. Like the "beauty industry" and the "fashion industry," such procedures are condemned as "unnecessary," "narcissistic," and "oppressive."

There is nothing new in these debates. Rational ascetic puritanism has consistently, since the Reformation, attacked the vices of adornment, and very old communitarian attitudes have always been suspicious of the luxuries of a cultivated life when measured against the imperatives of life-sustaining necessity. Yet to accept these attitudes means, for the humanistically inclined, to sacrifice the aesthetic qualities of elegance and beauty (however different societies and groups may define these). It means denying the aesthetic pleasure human beings get when they observe, or arrange, features of the body (hair, clothing, posture, figure, etc.) in a certain order or combination. The "lovers of appearances," of course, always run the risk of misjudging what is proportionate (to their age, build, circumstances, etc.) and thus fitting in appearance. In the case of the body, the risks are varied: all the way from simply looking silly to persons actually mutilating themselves. Yet to overdramatize such risks can also mean dismissing or denying the freedom that human beings experience when they observe or arrange the appearance of the body in (e.g.) consonant or beautiful forms. Appearances, arranged in certain proportions or in certain patterns, have the capacity to please (both the arranger and the spectator) on their own account, quite independently of life's necessities or society's functional imperatives. They are arranged, and are appreciated, for their own sake, and as such are emblematic of a kind of freedom. Of course—in part for the very reason that aesthetic pleasure involves a type of freedom—one cannot force aesthetic pleasure, and when any individual is made to participate in the culture of appearances against their will, this is certainly oppressive. For the rational ascetic or communitarian personality, the demands of appearances in modern urbane or cosmopolitan societies can be oppressive if the culture of appearances makes universalistic demands (the demands that everyone participate in the culture). But the same, equally, applies to the communitarian or rational ascetic. To generalize their cultures has similarly oppressive consequences.

Romantic

The fifth attitude toward the body is that of the romantic, for which the body is the site of transformation (or dissolution). Where the communitarian and the rationalist look for the assuredness of belonging or for the certainty engendered by the making of analytic distinctions and definitions, romantic representations of the body portray it in a state of change, of becoming. Romanticism is fascinated by the uncertainty or ambivalences of the body in transition. The romantic body is ever restless. It jumps, it sways; it is constantly on the point of change. Romantic representations of the body emphasize a certain haziness: the relentless succession of bodily states prevents any of them from attaining a relatively permanent or fixed shape. Of all the cultures of the body, it is the romantic that systematically challenges our conception of the identity of the body and the assumption that the body possesses relatively lasting or fixed features. The romantic emphasizes the human capacity to make and remake body states, in other words, the human capacity for self-determination. The romantic sees a key freedom in the ability of the self to escape, transgress, or redraw anything that gives the body shape or form or that encloses or limits it. The freedom of the romantic self is to be found, in other words, in its capacity to (constantly) redirect and redeploy bodily energies and activities.

In challenging conceptions of the identity of the body, the romantic often turns from the fixation on outward features (appearances) of the body to the ever-changing moods of the inward psychic life. For example, the use of hallucinogenic drugs in romantic subcultures of the 1960s was intended for the purpose of exploring the infinitely variable—and chaotic—inner world of the psyche. The romantic often treats the body as a vehicle of expression for inner states, in particular either ones that are postrational (ecstasy, intuition, speculation, and dreams) or pre-rational feelings states (e.g., fear) that are exaggerated and magnified into sublime states (of terror, horror, etc.). The romantic body, then, becomes a vehicle of passionate intensity, of constant highs and lows. As such, the romantic body lives in a state of constant agitation. It is "defined" only by its movement, or at the point of exhaustion of that movement, by its dissolution. The pathos of romantic culture is its inability to sustain indefinitely its attempt to escape any fixed or closed shape or state. On the one hand, this may lead to the "burn-out" of the romantic body, but also to a fascination with states of dissolution, with death, especially with the contemplation of suicide, with the "twilight" of life, with those ambiguous states in between life and death. For the romantic, dying has a morbid fascination. It offers, or insinuates, a distinctive form of "life"—one that is on the border, at the margins. It offers, in other words, the most ironic of all forms of "life." Like the *pharmakon*, which is both curative and poisonous, the dying person (like the dying culture) has lost life and yet is still living—a kind of death in life—and the irony of this, for the romantic, is unsurpassable and immensely seductive.

Postmodernism and the possibility of the contemporary state

What is of interest from a political point of view is not the fact that a plurality of cultures of the body exist but rather that they exist within common juridical and administrative (state) frameworks. Here we arrive at the paradox and conundrum of multicultural states. The paradox of these states is that they have a unitary legal/state framework, yet they contain, within that frame, a pluralism of normative (ethical) cultures. The conundrum of the multicultural states is: How, at all, are they possible?

When different cultural orientations clash, the temptation is to universalize (generalize) one or other cultural form—that is, legislatively, administratively, or juridically impose it on everyone. An exemplary (though by no means exceptional) case of this, in modern Western states, is the attempt by conservative communitarians to have abortions outlawed ("protect the unborn"), an attempt to entrench in law an ethical attitude that makes absolutely no sense in terms of any of the other cultural logics of modernity. But just as the ethical absolute of life cannot be generalized, neither can the goods of change, appearance, or rational asceticism. To attempt to do so is, invariably, to create oppressive universals.

Multicultural states are only possible where universal law is not used to destroy or disrupt cultural pluralism. To put it another way: universal law (law which is common to, or applicable to, all persons in the state) needs to be constructed to function to guarantee the access of individuals to the culture of their choice or disposition (with all its attendant freedoms and constraints, demands and benefits), and not to require the participation of all persons in one or other antinomical culture. There is little, in fact, that all persons in a modern state can and do share in common. We live, in other words, in a universe of minorities. As Agnes Heller observes, in an interesting discussion of this question, it is impossible, in the contemporary age, to assume that we can design the best possible way of life.[7] There are now, in fact, many ways of life, each of which is the "best possible" for those living it. The rationalist thinks that the ascetic regime is the "best possible"; the communitarian that the protective regime is the "best possible"; and so forth. The tragic aspect of modern Western, and especially European, societies has been the repeated attempts of those who thought their form of life was the "best possible" to impose it—if not by force, then by law, administration, or courts—on everyone else. Today, partly because of sober reflection on the disastrous results of these ambitions, this has become less legitimate. Less legitimate, though not illegitimate.

In many respects, what today is called "the postmodern condition" is both an acknowledgment of, and a retreat from, oppressive universals.[8] It is a sign, perhaps, that antinomical cultures may today be less prepared—or less able—to devour each other in the name of Reason, Humanity, God, or any other Transcendental or Quasi-transcendental subject. What comes of this can be only measured by the greater reluctance on the part of competing cultural forms to outlaw or prohibit each other, or plain terrorize each other, or else starve each other of public resources or recognition. This does not mean an end to tensions and disputes between the protagonists of antinomical cultural forms. All that it means is that it becomes (and properly so) more difficult for protagonists to use the common resources or regulation of the state to squeeze out their opponents. Take one example—the case of voluntary euthanasia. There is no doubting the fierceness and the depth of moral opposition to such a practice, yet today it has become almost as difficult to outlaw this practice (or at least find juries and courts willing to apply sanctions to it) as it is to compel such a practice. The reason for this is that, in modern societies, there are a number of radically contrasting or conflicting attitudes to the practice. Such (irresolvable) moral oppositions effectively undermine all attempts to turn ethical norms into legal imperatives. The communitarian may well condemn euthanasia. For the communitarian, life has an independent value. It is an end-in-itself. Life, therefore, should be prolonged as much as possible—even, some would argue, by the intervention of technological and scientific means—and certainly should not be cut short by human volition. Yet the communitarian cannot plausibly tell the rationalist or the romantic, who is terminally ill and suffering great and incapacitating pain, that their life should be medically prolonged because "life is sacred."

Life per se is not a good, or rather not the most important or central good, for the rationalist or the romantic. It is not an end in itself for the rationalist or the romantic. The rationalist judges his or her life in terms of productivity and contribution to society. The romantic judges life in terms of the opportunities it affords for adventure, for movement, and for change. When pain or disablement consistently confounds these orderings of life, the person concerned, possessed of all the facts, may well opt to request his or her doctor to cease medical treatment or even to administer a lethal drug. Of course, neither the romantic nor the rationalist may be able to fully comprehend or approve of each other's decision, and both will certainly be at odds with the communitarian. Even if the law is withdrawn from these debates, the debates themselves continue. What one regards as moral, the other will continue to regard as immoral or morally questionable. The protection or sanctity of life cannot be assimilated to a volitional death. The attitudes to the central questions of life and death remain at odds, fundamentally. And no political conciliation can, or even should, eliminate this irreducible *differend* between ethics.[9]

What, then, in the face of these moral antinomies and ambivalences is the function of the law? In a negative sense, we can say what the function of the law cannot be: it cannot be to generalize one ethic at the expense of another. What "the postmodern condition" assumes is the simultaneous existence of a number of "best possible" ways of life. Law, insofar as it is applicable to everyone in society, must be "neutral" between these different cultural worlds—that is, between the different cultural worlds that make up a modern cosmopolitan universe or cosmopolis. This does not mean that the law has no positive functions. It can still impose duties, but of a very specific kind. The legal duty of individuals, in a pluralistic universe, cannot be a legal duty toward themselves: the duty of individuals toward themselves in a pluralistic universe or cosmopolitan society is entirely a matter of their contingent ethic. All the law can properly prescribe are certain duties of individuals toward others: both general and specific duties that they have to respect and in certain ways help uphold the rights of others. If there is anything analogous to an *ius naturale* in modern societies, it is this: the rights of others are their rights to enter, participate in, and, if necessary, exit from the cultural form of their choice. Individuals, of course, can obstruct and interfere with the rights of others, and the positive role of the law in cosmopolitan settings is to reduce the spiral of obstruction and interference. The law has a particular responsibility to restrain those who would want to apply untoward pressure on, or force, others to abide by a certain ethical position. To be forced, intimidated, or pressured into a course of action or a decision by others because that action or decision conforms with *their* moral beliefs is quite at odds with the spirit of a cosmopolitan or polyvalent society. For this reason, the law, in such a society, properly defends rights: the rights of the communitarian to a fully protected life, of the romantic to an adventurous life, of the rationalist to an ascetic life, and so forth.

Of course, there will be situations when the rights of one person will conflict (sometimes tragically) with the rights or values of another person. What happens, e.g., when the communitarian doctor is asked by the rationalist or romantic patient to help them terminate their life? Such "hard cases" always threaten to disrupt the always precarious balance of a pluralistic universe, and *prudence* is what we must rely on to restore the balance when it is upset. Prudence may suggest that the doctor advise the patient to find another, more sympathetic, doctor, or else the patient reads the signs and does this for herself. Prudence may still fail us. Where there is no choice of doctor, the practical outcome will necessarily be tragic for either the doctor or the patient. But tragedy is not the norm of cosmopolitan societies. By definition, these are societies that are multifactorial or multidimensional, and collective (as opposed to individual) decision making and executive agencies are constituted, where they work well, as "empty spaces" that cannot be dominated by one or other cultural form but are really the place of intersection for different cultural logics in the society.[10]

In decisions or actions that have a public dimension—in matters of law and administration—agencies, again where they work well, don't force people constantly into sacrificial "either/or" choices; rather, they attempt to establish the balance of "both/and." A simple but illustrative example of this is the spending by the state on health care or care of the body. "Health" is by no means a simple entity; it is multidimensional. And no public allocation of resources to health is ever free of the countervailing demands of conflicting values. What properly constitutes the care of the body? Is it preventive health, or is it the methodical (medical-scientific) kind? Is it the stoical kind that emphasizes the independence of the self vis-à-vis the misfortunes and diseases of a life? Or is it the kind that prepares the self for life-changes? Or is it one that considers the way in which the presentation of self and body crucially affects a person's sense of esteem, well-being, and vitality? In the end, this is not a question just for administrators, just as the character of law in a pluralistic society is not just a question for lawyers. It is a political question. And as such it is properly the concern of citizens (singly or in associations), and their (parliamentary, congressional, etc.) representatives, acting and speaking in the public realm.

The domain of *the political* is the public sphere.[11] And it is in the public sphere that the countervailing claims of contestatory cultures can be put forward and elaborated. One of the great "modern myths," however, is the view that the public debate that ensues from this can and will lead to a rational consensus of views. Nobody is ever rationally convinced, one way or the other, as to what "ultimate attitudes" they hold fast to or relinquish, and debate is only ever persuasive in terms of these "ultimate attitudes." Public debate may, at the margins, convince adherents of a viewpoint of the need to make for themselves a more consistent case, or else it may bring them to honestly acknowledge those things which they cannot, within their own framework, account for. But this is always at the margins. What public debate really serves is something like the *ius gentium* of the Romans. The cultural logics of cosmopolitan societies are like the laws of different nations. The law of each nation is not, again except at the margins, going to change. The question for *ius gentium*, then, is how do these nations coexist civilly? The answer is that they do so through the prudent adjustment, or conciliation, of their claims.

Public debate is a process of adjustment, as cultural forms make room for others, and as the mentality of those in the public domain is enlarged, they come to acknowledge and take account of other viewpoints. The denizens of each cultural form stake a claim in the public domain—a claim for a certain "best possible" moral world to be recognized in law and for a "fair share" of public resources to sustain that form of life for the benefit of its (voluntary) adherents and participants. These claims are also, more often than not, a critique of the overextension of competing cultures, their disregard of the claimant culture, or their (relative) monopolization of public resources. Such critiques represent the attempt to set boundaries or limits between cultural formations. When this political process is successful—and there are never any guarantees of this—neither one or other cultural logic will dominate, nor will one or other necessarily disappear. Rather, there will be a civil or "working relationship" that allows each their own institutions, spaces, and constituencies, yet at the same time demands of each a sense of, and respect for, being part of a more complex, multidimensional whole.

Notes

1   For a discussion of the centrality of culture, and an elaboration of a "culturalogical" perspective, see the work of Johann P. Arnason. Of particular interest are his "Culture and Imaginary Significations," *Thesis Eleven* 22 (1989), pp. 25–45, and "Civilization, Culture and Power: Reflections on Norbert Elias' Genealogy of the West," *Thesis Eleven* 24 (1989), pp. 66–70.

2   The most interesting discussion of the emergence of the idea of "society" is that offered by Hannah Arendt. In particular, see *On Revolution* (Harmondsworth, Penguin, 1973), chap. 2, and *The Human Condition* (Chicago, University of Chicago Press, 1958), chap. 2. Other, also interesting, observations on this question are offered by Michel Foucault in *The History of Sexuality*, vol. 1 (Harmondsworth, Penguin, 1981), parts 4–5. Much of Foucault's analysis of biopolitics, though, does little more than cover ground already traversed by Arendt.

3   The typology of feelings that I advance in this article draws on the typology of feelings proposed by Agnes Heller in *A Theory of Feelings* (The Netherlands, Van Gorcum Assen, 1979), chap. 2.

4   Arendt, *Human Condition*.

5   Heller, *Theory of Feelings*, chap. 2.

6   Arendt, in a very interesting defense of this attitude, argues for the importance of appearances to human beings against the philosophical traditions that value essence over appearance. See the first section of the first volume of her *The Life of the Mind* (New York, Harcourt, 1978).

7   Agnes Heller, *Beyond Justice* (Oxford, Basil Blackwell, 1987), chap. 5. See also Heller, "Rationality and Democracy," in *The Power of Shame* (London, Routledge, 1985); Heller, "Freedom and Happiness in Kant's Political Philosophy" and "Rights, Modernity, Democracy" in *Can Modernity Survive?* (Oxford, Polity, 1990).

8   There have been many attempts to describe the postmodern condition. The best of these attempts are to be found in the work of Jean-François Lyotard, Agnes Heller, Ferenc Feher,

and Charles Jencks. See Lyotard's *The Postmodern Condition* (Manchester, Manchester University Press, 1984), and "Universal History and Cultural Differences," "Judiciousness in Dispute, or Kant after Marx" and "The Sign of History," in Andrew Benjamin, ed., *The Lyotard Reader* (Oxford, Blackwell, 1989); Agnes Heller and Ferenc Feher, *The Postmodern Political Condition* (Oxford, Polity, 1988), in particular Feher's essays, "The Status of Postmodernity" and "Between Relativism and Fundamentalism: Hermeneutics as Europe's Mainstream Political and Moral Tradition," in Heller and Feher, *The Grandeur and Twilight of Radical Universalism* (New Brunswick, N.J., Transaction Books, 1991); Charles Jencks, *Post-modernism* (New York, Rizzoli, 1987).

9   The term *differend* comes from Jean-François Lyotard, *The Differend* (Manchester, Manchester University Press, 1988).

10   The term *empty spaces* was proposed by Claude Lefort. See his *The Political Forms of Modern Society* (Oxford, Polity, 1987), and *Democracy and Political Theory* (Oxford, Polity, 1988). For some interesting reflections, and elaborations, on Lefort's idea, see Dick Howard, *The Politics of Critique* (London, Macmillan, 1989).

11   On the concept of the political, see Howard, *Politics of Critique* and *Defining the Political* (London, Macmillan, 1989).

Whose body? Feminist views on reproductive technology

Max Charlesworth

Developments in feminism

The feminist voice—or better, feminist voices—have played a significant part in the debate over the moral and social implications of the new reproductive technologies. Since women are affected by in vitro fertilization and other forms of reproductive technology in a much more direct and momentous way than men, it is altogether to be expected that they will be major contributors to the discussion. To some degree, it is true, the male experience in reproductive technology has been neglected: men in an infertile situation often choose to undergo difficult and recurrent surgery to remedy their infertility and, so it has been said, "male emotions, desires and anger (apropos infertility) are equal to that of the female, albeit expressed differently."[1] Nevertheless, it remains true that it is women who usually have to undergo the major medical procedures and who bear the children brought into being by the new birth technologies. It is their bodies which are, so to speak, in contention.

When women speak about these technologies then their views deserve special attention. The fact is, however, that they speak in a variety of different voices. Carol Gilligan's influential book *In a Different Voice*, argues that each woman has a distinctive experience and a distinctive expression of that experience.[2] However, over the last twenty years feminist responses to the new birth technologies have undergone a radical series of changes and there is now a genuine "pluralism" of voices and views. They are, no doubt, still distinctively feminist views and bear a "family resemblance" to each other, but they are also very different from each other.

Some feminist thinkers have traced these developments to demographic and social changes within the body of middle-class women over the last twenty years. Thus, three English feminists—Lynda Birke, Susan Himmelweit, and Gail Vines—observe that "in the early 1970s, when the current wave of feminism began, most of the women involved in the movement had had their children and were searching for other means of fulfilment in their lives, or had not had children and were not yet having to face the issue of whether they ever would choose to be mothers. Both groups saw it important to prove that women did not have to be seen only in terms of their reproductive abilities. For both groups, reproductive freedom meant freedom *from* reproduction." However, these authors go on, some women of this group are now more interested in having children because they are growing older—women who were in their twenties in the 1970s can no longer delay childbearing and have to make a decision—and because of changes in the political climate. "Feminism," they say, "is no longer for many women the totally absorbing activity and form of self-definition it once was. Feminists, like others, may be turning inwards to rear children, perhaps as the only social contribution to make in a period of reaction and political quiescence." As a result, they conclude, "Babies themselves, not just the limitations they impose on their mothers' lives, have after a period of near oblivion, become a matter of interest to the women's movement. And this has led a few feminists to experience problems with their own infertility, and even more to take an interest in the issues surrounding pregnancy and child-birth, including infertility and its treatment."[3]

Quite apart from these factors, there has been a natural movement of critical revisionism within feminism. All revolutionary movements, whether they are political or religious or philosophical, usually begin with absolute and uni-lateral positions; they then pass through a reflective and critical revisionist phase to a more pluralist position characterized by the emergence and accep-tance of differing perspectives and interpretive frameworks. This kind of de-velopment is clearly observable in many religious movements and in philo-sophical movements like Marxism and Freudianism, and it is not surprising that it is now appearing within feminism. One could, in fact, apply to the feminist movement as a whole the observation by Carol Gilligan that personal cognitive maturity involves "changes in thinking that mark the transition from a belief that knowledge is absolute and answers clearly right or wrong to an understanding of the contextual relativity of both truth and choice."[4]

Some may see this as a sign of incoherence and confusion within the feminist position, but I for one certainly do not. In my view it is an index of maturity in any movement—religious, political, artistic, or feminist—that it is ready to eschew a strictly monolithic position and tolerate, even welcome, a variety of views and positions. Pluralism is a sign of vitality and strength and not of exhaustion and weakness and confusion.

Rejection of reproductive technology

In the early 1970s a number of feminist thinkers welcomed the advent of the new reproductive technologies as a means of liberation for women from the tyranny of their biological nature which condemned them to pregnancy and childbearing and -rearing. For example, American writer Shulamith Firestone argued in her book *The Dialectic of Sex*[5] that artificial reproduction would eventually allow women to escape the "barbaric" state of pregnancy. This in turn would allow women to overcome their oppressed social position which is a direct consequence of their biology. Firestone's position, and that of other "first-wave" feminists who shared her views, rested on a naively optimistic view of technology as though it were value-neutral and could be used at will by women for their own liberatory ends. In the 1970s and 1980s, however, the critique of this view of technology by thinkers such as Langdon Winner, Jacques Ellul, and others, showed how deeply the various forms of technology are already pervaded by sociopolitical values and how difficult it is to make technology serve the cause of human liberation. The technopessimism, as one may call it, that emerged from this critique combined with the environmentalist movement to show that in many cases the technology that was supposed to free us from the determinisms of nature in fact enslaved us further.

This critical and pessimistic attitude to technology was taken over in the 1980s by a number of feminist thinkers vis-à-vis the new reproductive technologies. The older, naively optimistic, view that these technologies were an instrument of liberation for women (like the new contraceptive and abortifacient technologies) was rejected, and they were now seen as a means of male oppression of women under the guise of liberating them. The technologies, it was said, involved women's bodies being used by male scientists for research and, at a deeper level, they were an attempt to deprive women of power over their most distinctive capacity, reproduction, and make it subject to male control.

A further element in this argument is that infertile women are led to submit themselves to this kind of scientific exploitation because of the "pro-natalist" pressures of our society making them see reproduction as bound up with their identity as women. A quasi-Marxist idea of false consciousness was also introduced in order to explain many women's desire to have children: they may really think they have such a desire, but they are not aware that it is a false desire induced in them by society—it is, to use a modish (and misleading) term, "socially constructed." Further, by satisfying their own self-interested personal wishes to have a child through in vitro fertilization (IVF) they are conniving in the larger exploitation of women and betraying a lack of feminine conscious-ness. As Mara Mies has said, "any woman who is prepared to have a child manufactured for her by a fame- and money-greedy biotechnician must know that in this way she is not only fulfilling herself in an individual, often egoistic wish to have a baby, but also surrendering yet another part of the autonomy of the female sex over childbearing to the technopatriarchs."[6]

It was argued that this false consciousness on the part of women who resort to IVF and other forms of reproductive technology in turn provides a basis for legitimate paternalism since women in this situation do not really know what is for their own good or for the common good of women as a whole and they have to be prevented, for their own good and the good of women as a class, from us-ing the new reproductive technologies. Another feature of this position was its tendency to invent what might be called Orwellian scenarios where the future horrors of reproductive technology—mechanical wombs, using neo-morts as fetal incubators, gendercide through sex selection—were imaginatively con-jured up. The most dramatic of these scenarios was the "reproductive brothel" of Gena Corea: "While sexual prostitutes sell vagina, rectum and mouth, re-productive prostitutes will sell other body parts: womb, ovaries, eggs."[7] This general position was espoused by feminist thinkers in the early 1980s such as Gena Corea and Christine Overall,[8] and one of its main expressions is to be found in the FINRRAGE movement (the Feminist International Network of Resistance to Reproductive and Genetic Technology) associated in Australia with the names of Robyn Rowland, Renate Klein, and others. One of the curious features of this movement is that it has found itself in coalition not just, as one would expect, with the Green movement but also with conservative Catholics and fundamentalist Christians who are in most other respects (e.g., on abortion and female homosexuality) totally at odds with the radical feminist position. Thus, for example, the Vatican rejection of IVF was welcomed by some members of FINRRAGE, and they have also found common cause with conserva-tive Christian views on embryo experimentation and surrogate motherhood.

Of course this does not constitute an objection to this position; what is more difficult to explain, however, is why the technology of IVF and the other forms of artificial procreation were singled out for opposition. After all, the con-traceptive pill and other means of contraception are forms of technology, as are the various forms of abortifacients. These kinds of technology were also part of male paternalistic science and involved the intervention of men in the process of reproduction and the use of women in scientific experimentation, but they were not seen by these feminists as attempts to deprive women of their re-productive powers. Contraceptive and abortifacient technologies, which en-abled women not to have children, were seen as conducive to women's libera-tion (although there have been feminist criticisms of male insensitivities in contraceptive research and development). Again, women who used contracep-tive and abortifacient technologies were not presumed to be victims of false consciousness or of letting the feminist cause down; they were deemed in need of paternalistic advice and direction (even legal coercion). They were, it seems to have been assumed, capable of autonomous decision making about con-traceptive and abortifacient technology in a way in which they were not capa-ble of freely and autonomously choosing for themselves about reproductive technology.

Surrogacy and embryo experimentation

It is worthwhile to look at the arguments used by proponents of this position against surrogacy and embryo experimentation. With regard to the question of surrogate motherhood, some feminists of this persuasion have argued that it is impossible for a woman to choose freely and autonomously to act as a surro-gate mother and to bear a child for another woman. There are two variants of this argument: first, that surrogate motherhood is *of itself* so exploitative of women that it cannot be freely chosen, any more than a person could freely choose to be a slave; second, that *in the present social situation* it is not possible for a woman freely and autonomously to choose to bear a child for another. The first variant is represented by Christine Overall who claims that "there is a real moral danger in the type of conceptual framework that presents surrogate motherhood as even a possible freely chosen alternative for women."[9] The second is represented by Susan Dodds and Karen Jones who argue that in our present social situation "it is unlikely that many women can make an autono-mous choice to enter into a surrogacy contract which would compel them to surrender the child at birth."[10] Dodds and Jones do not argue that surrogacy as such cannot be chosen as an option by a woman, but that in the present situation of society where women are oppressed and exploited, they cannot make such decisions. This in turn legitimates paternalistic action by the state to prevent women choosing to bear children for other women.

> If the world were different, a policy of making surrogacy contracts illegal
> might not be necessary. If surrogacy agreements were clearly not exploit-

ative offers, and if monitoring occurred to ensure that a decision to become a surrogate reflected and protected a woman's autonomy, then,
perhaps, such agreements would be viable. However, that is not the present situation, and so surrogacy contracts must become not only unen-
forceable, but, as they pay insufficient regard for the resultant child and
tend to risk commodifying both women and children, illegal.[11]

This strongly paternalistic attitude goes together, in some feminist arguments,
with a critique of an "individualistic" concept of rights and of moral "liber-
tarianism" based on the principle of autonomy. To the objection that feminist
views of contraception and abortion rely on the right of a woman to choose
whether or not to have a child and on the autonomy of women in respect of
their control over their own bodies, one answer is that abortion is often a
socially responsible act and is not justified solely in terms of the individualistic
right of a woman to do what she wants to do with her own body. As it has been
put: abortion is "an act of social responsibility with respect to family formation."[12] It is not clear, however, why the use of abortifacient technology in order
not to have a child *is* an "act of social responsibility" and why the use of
reproductive technology in order to *have* a child is *not* socially responsible.

   With regard to embryo experimentation, some feminists subscribing to the
position we have been describing oppose such experimentation not because the
IVF embryo is seen as a human person with the same right to life as a fully
formed human person, but because embryos come from the ova "harvested"
from women's bodies and the latter become experimental "sites" for reproductive scientists. The use of superovulatory drugs and invasive surgical techniques
also mean that women become experimental "fodder." As it has been put by
Robyn Rowland, "The feminist position on embryo experimentation does not
recognise the embryo as a separate human entity. It makes both women and the
social context central to its position. Few protagonists in the embryo experimentation debate ask where the embryos came from. They come from eggs.
And where do the eggs come from? They come from women's bodies."[13] These
feminists are also concerned that this kind of experimentation will lead to sex
selection of early embryos with the consequence that female embryos will be
systematically eliminated in favor of male embryos. In other words, we will end
with a form of "gendercide."

   In general, this feminist position claims that "IVF is an unsuccessful technology that threatens the freedom and the well-being of women, and that only a

few white, middle-class heterosexual couples will benefit from IVF, along with the shareholders of genetic engineering companies. A woman's participation in reproductive technology is thus the result of conforming to the whims of male domination."[14]

New feminist views

This stringent critique of reproductive technology was, perhaps, the dominant view in "second-wave" feminist thinking through the 1980s and still retains a good deal of influence. There are now signs that the absolute rejection of reproductive technology is being critically reassessed by some recent feminists, however. These thinkers reject the naive optimism of early feminists like Firestone and recognize with Corea that the new technology is not value-neutral but is in fact pervaded by certain technocratic values, and that there are real dangers of it being used against women in an exploitative way. At the same time, they argue that the reproductive technologies can be used to help women achieve liberation if they are able to control those technologies for their own purposes. If the "pro-choice" principle governs women's access to the new forms of contraception and to improved ways of abortion—both brought about by medical technology—why should it not govern women's access to IVF and the other forms of birth technology, provided that there is a real choice for the women concerned?

A good example of this development in feminist thinking is the recently published *Tomorrow's Child: Reproductive Technology in the 1990s* by three well-known English feminists. In their preface, Birke et al. characterize the FINRRAGE position as being dominated by fear: "fear that what we are witnessing is a takeover by scientists of women's role in reproduction, and fear that we are moving towards a dehumanised (and defeminised) technological future. The position is one of total resistance to scientific and male control of reproductive processes, by a complete rejection of the new technologies." Against this, they affirm the primacy of the feminist principle "that women should be able to choose whether or not to bear a child": "We feel that women, and women alone, should be the ones to make the choice."[15]

At the same time, Birke et al. adopt an attitude of healthy skepticism toward some of the more extreme reproductive scenarios (the possibility of ectogenesis and the mechanical womb, the use of ova donation and embryo transfer to create Corea's and Dworkin's "reproductive brothel"). They also question the version of Murphy's Law which a good deal of previous feminist thinking has invoked: if a biotechnological development is theoretically possible, it is likely actually to occur and it is bound to be bad for women. This is, the authors argue, to adopt an unduly pessimistic view in that it assumes that women are unable to resist pressures from male medical technocrats and are incapable of taking control of the technology themselves (as has happened to some extent in ordinary birthing practices).

In the conclusion to their book the authors set out a number of "feminist principles" which supplement the "pro choice" principle and provide a social and political dimension to their discussion. Reproductive politics, they say, must find ways of changing the arrangements for reproduction in our society which are oppressive to women, and of enabling women to carry out effectively their reproductive choices. A similar view has been taken by the American feminist philosopher Mary Anne Warren, who argues that while "the costs and risks of IVF treatments to the female patient are substantial . . . they are not known to be so great as to clearly outweigh the potential benefits, in every case." There are physical and social dangers for women in reproductive technology, but women can by various means attempt to contain these dangers rather than seek to eliminate the new technologies altogether. They must also work to gain more control of the technologies. Warren says that "it is too soon to conclude that this new reproductive technology will not serve women's interest. If women and other underprivileged groups can gain a larger presence in the medical and research professions, and if suitable modes of regulation can be implemented, then the new reproductive technologies may provide more benefits than dangers."[16]

Another feminist philosopher, Laura Purdy, also argues against the position that surrogacy is necessarily opposed to women's best interests:

> [That] surrogacy reduces rather than promotes women's autonomy may be true under some circumstances, but there are good grounds for thinking that it can also enhance autonomy. It also remains to be shown that the practice systematically burdens women, or one class of women. In principle, the availability of new choices can be expected to nourish rather than stunt women's lives, so long as they retain control over their bodies and their lives. The claim that contracted pregnancy destroys women's individuality and constitutes alienated labour, as Christine Overall argues, depends not only a problematic Marxist analysis, but on the assumption that other jobs available to women are seriously less alienating.[17]

An optimistic view of the "procreative technologies" and of surrogate mother-hood is also put forward by American legal scholar Lisa C. Ikemoto, who argues that they "increase availability of choice, thereby increasing the opportunity for women to achieve autonomy through decision-making. This in turn advances sexual equality." Ikemoto goes on:

> Some feminists have disparaged the institution of motherhood by stating that it prevents women from achieving equality. Other women, including feminists, see it in more positive terms. Surrogate motherhood gives infer-tile women or women who fear transmitting deleterious genes a chance to enjoy the childrearing aspect of motherhood. No less important is that surrogate motherhood constitutes a vehicle for a woman to help another woman in a uniquely feminine way, by carrying her child.[18]

A different kind of argument about surrogacy has been proposed by Austra-lian sociologist and feminist Sharyn L. Roach Anleu. She states that the distinc-tion between commercial and altruistic surrogacy is neither self-evident nor natural, but in fact reflects and reinforces gender norms. Altruistic surrogacy is seen as belonging to the private domestic sphere where relationships "are supposed to be based on affection and emotion which are private, irrational sentiments, thereby inappropriate subjects for legal regulation." It is therefore more accepted, or at least not so sharply condemned, as commercial surrogacy. Roach Anleu concludes:

> In a sense surrogacy is an extension of the kinds of nurturing related activities women have always performed, such as child rearing, which have not always been recognised as compensatable work, but treated as result-ing from natural female emotions and instincts. Paid surrogacy breaks the myth of the maternal instinct; not only can women have babies and give them away, but they can also enter into a contract that actually rewards them for having babies. Anything less than that is exploitation because the notion of altruistic choice is socially constructed and reinforces gender norms; payment for services questions gender norms."[19]

Birke et al. make the same point about the private/public distinction. Sur-rogacy, they say, offends people, because it represents "an overstepping of the boundaries between public and private, the introduction of the public way of getting people to do things by paying them money, into an activity which is supposed to remain within the private sphere." Feminists, they conclude, "should be suspicious of such distinctions; the division between public and private has on the whole been oppressive to women and has been used to keep them out of the public arena."[20]

With regard to the issue of embryo experimentation Karen Dawson and Beth Gaze accept the claim of Robyn Rowland and others that the present debate is focused too much on the embryo, without taking into account the woman who supplies the ovum and who is the subject of research. However, they say, "the separation of embryo research from the woman's treatment has led to a situation where women undergoing IVF treatment continue to accept the transfer of potentially defective embryos and the possibility of miscarriage, therapeutic abortion, or giving birth to a child with congenital abnormalities, because of their commitment to the goal of having a child." If this situation is to be remedied and women protected some embryo research and experimentation must be carried out.[21]

In a recent essay Mary Anne Warren claims that women are able to make free and autonomous decisions about donating embryos for research and experimentation. At the same time, she lays down a number of prescriptions to be observed by reproductive scientists and technologists in order to ensure that genuinely informed consent be possible by the women in IVF programs.[22] What is essential is that IVF, embryo experimentation, and all the other procedures connected with IVF should as far as possible be in the control of women. Warren uses very much the same kind of argumentation in a study of sex selection and the danger of "gendercide": "Sex selection is not always sexist, socially harmful, or disrespectful of the child as an end in itself. Its sexism and its potential for harm are very much a function of how it is done, why it is done, and the social context. That being the case, universal condemnation seems inappropriate, and regulation preferable, at least in the first instance, to prohibition."[23]

The "third-wave" feminists just mentioned do not constitute a "school" or a "movement"; nevertheless, there are certain common features in their approaches to the new reproductive technologies. First, they are critical of any absolute and unilateral rejection of the new technologies and of the technopessimism that sees the technologies as beyond any kind of control by women. Control, they suggest, is what is needed and not condemnation or prohibition. At the same time, they recognize the difficulties in the way of achieving informed consent and control by women. This group is also skeptical of the Orwellian future scenarios imagined by Corea and others of the FINRRAGE group, and they are critical of the paternalistic attitudes of the same group which, as has been said, are "insulting" to infertile women.[24] As an older feminist thinker, Janet Radcliffe Richards, has put it: "It is too dangerous to try to 'free' women who are regarded as conditioned by forcing them to do what prevailing feminist ideology presumes they must want, because with that method there is always the danger of ignoring women's real wishes. They may not be conditioned at all."[25]

A different "phenomenological" perspective on these issues is provided by an American feminist and nurse, Margarete Sandelowski.[26] Basing her observations on extensive interview data with infertile women, Sandelowski describes the painfully ambivalent position of such women vis-à-vis the feminist movement. As noted before, they are judged by some feminists to be victims of false consciousness and of being self-interestedly dismissive of the common good of women. Sandelowski replies to these charges by emphasizing the legitimacy of individual women's experience of infertility and of their desires to have children with the assistance of technology.

> The infertile woman, here and now, forces those of us who care for her to deal with a distinctively feminist moral dilemma: how to engage an individual woman's concrete situation in its immediacy while engaging the condition of women as a social group. Feminists call for social rather than individual solutions to the problem that technological and other controversial solutions (such as surrogacy) for infertility pose for women and for feminist theory and action, but infertility itself is experienced individually. . . . The first social solution to the problem with no nice feminist answer is for feminists neither to minimize the painful reality of infertility nor to trivialise the desire to conceive and bear a child. We do not have to deny the infertile woman's agency to be vigilant of the consequences for women of technological developments in reproduction. We do not have to question the infertile woman's right to choose the solutions to infertility available to her to affirm any woman's right to reproductive freedom. We do not have to suspect the infertile woman's desire for a child of her "own" (genetically, gestationally), or a child who might have been her own, to celebrate the value of all children or to protect birth mothers from being forced to relinquish their children. We do have to make a comfortable place for her at the centre of our passionate debates."[27]

A "feminist ethics"?

A number of feminist thinkers have canvased the possibility of a "feminist ethics"—that is, a view of ethics that would be based on women's distinctive experience as women and on feminist values, and which would have a specifically feminist perspective. Delineating that experience and specifying those values is, however, not an easy task. There is a form of "vulgar feminism" (analogous to vulgar Marxism) which likes to make a wish list of desirable and admirable human qualities—sensitivity, intuitiveness, feeling, caring, nurturing, and so on—and a contrary list of undesirable human qualities (abstractness, rationalism, manipulativeness, and aggressiveness) and which then arbitrarily dubs the former to be the preserve of "the feminine" and the latter the preserve of "the masculine." This kind of enterprise involves massive simplifications and arbitrary classifications and dichotomies which totally neglect individual differences, as well as class and culture differences. In a sense it is essentialism (as though there were an essential and eternal "feminine") and the abstract spirit (supposedly the peculiar vice of male thinkers) run riot. It also betrays a considerable ignorance of history. Despite the Western European historical record of male domination and aggression, there is also a countervailing history of emphasis on the aesthetic, personal interiority, the "heart" as against cold reason or the "mystical." After all, the Romantic movement of the eighteenth and nineteenth centuries also powerfully emphasized the values of the realm of what one feminist calls "the personal-private, emotional, interiorized, particular, individuated, intimate"[28] in opposition to the scientific and technological spirit of the age. Those values cannot therefore be seen as the exclusive preserve of women and be the basis for a "feminist ethics".

In one sense, of course, a feminist perspective or point of view will make a difference to the kinds of ethical issues that are seen as central very much as a religious perspective will make a difference to one's view of ethical paradigms. Thus, American philosopher Annette Baier juxtaposes what she calls an "ethics of love," which she sees as a typically feminine approach, to an "ethics of obligation," which she sees as a typically male approach. Most ethical theories, she claims, are preoccupied with the concept of obligation and duty and "give only hand waves concerning our proper attitudes to our children, the ill, to our relatives, friends and lovers." Baier goes on to discuss the central place in ethics of what she calls "appropriate trust": "A very complex network of a great variety of sorts of trust structures our moral relationships with our fellows, and if there is a main support to this network it is the trust we place in those who respond to the trust of new members of the moral community, namely to children, and to prepare them for new forms of trust." [29] These trust relationships, she suggests, are an important part of women's experience, and they provide a profoundly different ethical perspective.

There is, of course, a good deal in this but it cannot be pressed too far. As Baier admits, there have been in the history of ethics a number of theories elaborated by male moral philosophers which have attempted to emphasize experiences and values (of trust, friendship, and love, for example) which cannot be subsumed under the concepts of obligation and duty. The present anti-Kantian and pro-Aristotelian trend in Anglo-American ethics is a case in point.

Some have gone further than claiming that there is a distinctive feminist ethical *perspective* and have suggested, more radically, that there can be a distinctive feminist ethical *methodology*, as though the canons of inquiry that apply in ethical discussion could be distinctively feminine and, in a sense, available only to women. Thus, it has been argued that women's experience and their ways of knowing and loving and their "discourse" cannot be accommodated within what Irigaray calls a "patriarchal logic."[30] In my view, however, this is an incoherent position since the case that there is such a "feminist ethics," with its own distinctive methodological and epistemological canons, has to be argued in terms of commonly accepted "gender-free" norms of rationality (in the same way as Marxists who argue that the prevailing view of rationality is "ideologically" shaped by the class structures of our society, have nevertheless to argue their case in terms of that view of rationality). There is no doubt that our conceptions of the norms of rationality (objectivity and verifiability, for example) can be influenced by social and gender factors and that they continually need to be critically purified, but that does not mean that the norms are completely *determined* by those factors and that there is no way of appealing to canons of rationality (in science, philosophy, or ethics) that transcend both social and gender determination, and equally no way of distinguishing between truth and ideology.

The claim by some feminist thinkers that opposition to certain feminist philosophical positions can be explained (and dismissed) as being due to male patriachalist modes of reasoning is similar to the claim by some Freudians that opposition to Freud's philosophical and scientific position can be explained in psychoanalytical terms. But both are, surely, absurd. In a recent essay an English feminist philosopher, Sara Coakley, has argued for a recognition of "global principles" (trans-gender) in ethics: "As the heady shift to postmodern relativism becomes an attractive philosophical option for increasing numbers of feminists, we may well question whether the Enlightenment demand for global principles in ethics (as opposed to local political agendas) can be lightly discarded when what we surely must still dream of is an 'abolition of the sex class system tout court.' "[31]

The hope that a feminist ethics (of this radical kind) is possible is also a dangerous one for women to adopt in that if it is taken seriously it completely surrenders the field of rational discourse in ethics to men. A great deal can be done, and has been done by feminists to question and modify the rules and canons of the ethical and bioethical discourse to ensure that male biases and distortions are corrected so that they are more sensitive to women's experience and concerns. But it is another thing entirely to wish to invent a quite different ethical discourse with methodological rules of its own.

There are analogies here with the ideas of some feminist philosophers of science who have questioned the gender neutrality of "objectivity" and other central criteria of the "scientific."[32] Some have concluded that science is irretrievably a masculine project and that the only alternatives for feminists are either to reject science altogether or to envisage a radically new form of science with different criteria of the "scientific." With regard to the first alternative, Evelyn Fox Keller, an American philosopher of science, has argued that it is "suicidal." So she says: "By rejecting objectivity as a masculine ideal it simultaneously lends its voice to an enemy chorus and dooms women to residing outside the Realpolitik male modern culture: it exacerbates the very problem it wishes to solve."[33] Again, with respect to the second alternative, the same author has this to say: "The assumption that science can be replaced de novo reflects a view of science as pure social product, owing obedience to moral and political pressure from without. In this extreme relativism, science dissolves into ideology; any emancipatory function of modern science is negated, and the arbitration of truth recedes into the political domain." Fox Keller proposes instead "the reclamation, from within science, of science as a human instead of a masculine project, and the renunciation of the division of emotional and intellectual labour that maintains science as a male preserve."[34] One could easily, and fruitfully, transpose what Keller says here about "feminist science" to the fields of ethics in general and to bioethics in particular. In effect this is the theme of a recent essay by American feminist Sidney Callahan;[35] while questioning the possibility of a gender-based ethics, Callahan makes the point that the experiences of women give them uniquely different data to bring to the process of moral reflection.

Summing up

In this essay I have for the most part presented the various forms of feminist thinking about the new reproductive technologies in a more or less descriptive way. As I remarked at the beginning there is now a genuine pluralism of feminist views about the issues raised by IVF and other modes of artificial procreation and the debate between the different feminist positions is an interesting and fruitful one.

To a large degree those positions reflect those taken up in the general debate about the nature and meaning of human technology with technopessimists at one extreme and technooptimists at the other.[36] The technopessimists emphasize that technology is never neutral or value-free and that it is difficult, indeed almost impossible, to control and use it for human purposes. The technooptimists on the other hand emphasize that technology enables us to escape from the determinisms and "fatalisms" of nature and can easily be made to serve the cause of human liberation. In my view, the feminist debate over reproductive technology points to a middle way between those two extremes.

In a sense, the human body is a place where nature and technology meet. On the one hand there are the physiological and genetic and biological "givens"— elements of bodily "facticity," to use Sartre's term. On the other hand, the biological processes and dispositions of the body have to be endowed with human meaning and significance by what the Greeks called *techne* and which we have usually translated as "art." In this view, technology is an extension or prolongation of the capacities and possibilities of the human body.

In analogous ways, the new reproductive technologies or "arts" can extend or prolong the natural biological processes of human reproduction and, despite the dangers of hubris and misuse, open up new human possibilities in the bodies of both women and men.

Notes

This chapter is an expanded version of a section of my book, *Bioethics in a Liberal Society* (Cambridge, Cambridge University Press, 1993).

1 Professor Colin D. Matthews in *Surrogacy: Biomedical Dilemmas in the 1990s* (Adelaide, Dietrich Bonhoeffer International Institute for Bioethical Studies, 1990), p. 4.

2 Carol Gilligan, *In a Different Voice: Psychological Theory and Women's Development* (Cambridge, Mass., Harvard University Press, 1982). For criticisms of Gilligan, see Onora O'Neill and Marth Nussbaum, "Justice, Gender and International Boundaries," in Martha Nussbaum and Amartyn Sen, eds., *The Quality of Life* (Oxford, Clarendon Press, 1993).

3 Lynda Birke, Susan Himmelweit, and Gail Vines, *Tomorrow's Child: Reproductive Technology in the 1990s* (London, Virago Press, 1990), pp. 3–4.

4 Gilligan, *In a Different Voice*, p. 166.

5 Shulamith Firestone, *The Dialectic of Sex* (New York, Jonathan Cape, 1971).

6   Mara Mies, "Do We Need All This? A Call against Genetic Engineering and Reproductive Technology," in Patricia Spallone and Deborah Steinberg, eds., *Made to Order: The Myth of Reproductive and Genetic Progress* (New York, Oxford University Press, 1987).

7   Gena Corea, *The Mother Machine* (New York, Harper and Row, 1982), p. 39.

8   Corea, *Mother Machine*; Christine Overall, *Ethics and Human Reproduction* (London, Allen and Unwin, 1983).

9   Overall, *Ethics and Human Reproduction*, p. 125.

10 Susan Dodds and Karen Jones, "Surrogacy and Autonomy," *Bioethics* 3, no. 1 (1989), p. 13.

11 Ibid., p. 17.

12 See Heather Dietrich, "Dissenting View, Surrogacy Report" (Adelaide, National Bioethics Consultative Committee, 1990), p. 62.

13 Robyn Rowland, "Making Women Visible in the Embryo Experimentation Debate," *Bioethics* 1, no. 2 (1987), p. 5.

14 Karen Dawson, "Human Embryo Experimentation: A Background Paper and Select Bibliography" (Adelaide, National Bioethics Consultative Committee, 1990), p. 32. This is not Dawson's own position.

15 Birke et al., *Tomorrow's Child*, p. x.

16 Mary Ann Warren, "IVF and Women's Interests," *Bioethics* 2, no. 1 (1988), pp. 53–54.

17 Laura Purdy, "Surrogate Mothering: Exploitation or Empowerment?" *Bioethics* 3, no. 1 (1989), p. 24.

18 Lisa C. Ikemoto, "Providing Protection for Collaborative, Noncoital Reproduction: Surrogate Motherhood and Other New Procreative Technologies, and the Right of Intimate Association," *Rutgers Law Review* 40 (1988), pp. 1302–1303.

19 Sharyn L. Roach Anleu, "Reinforcing Gender Norms: Commercial and Altruistic Surrogacy," *Acta Sociologica* 33, 1 (1990), pp. 70, 72.

20 Birke et al., *Tomorrow's Child*, pp. 266–267.

21 Karen Dawson and Beth Gaze, "Who Is the Subject of the Research?" in Peter Singer and Helga Kuhse et al., eds., *Embryo Experimentation* (Cambridge, Cambridge University Press, 1990).

22 Mary Ann Warren, "Is IVF a Threat to Women's Autonomy?" In *Embryo Experimentation*, pp. 125–140.

23 Mary Ann Warren, "A Reply to Holmes on Gendercide," *Bioethics* 1, no. 2 (1987), p. 198. See also Warren's book, *Gendercide: The Implications of Sex Selection* (Totowa, N.J., Rowman and Allanheld, 1985). See also Marlene Gerber Fried, ed., *From Abortion to Reproductive Freedom: Transforming a Movement* (Boston, South End Press, 1990), especially the essay by Kathryn Kolbert, "Developing a Reproductive Rights Agenda for the 1990s."

24 Birke et al., *Tomorrow's Child*, p. 310.

25 Janet Radcliffe Richards, *The Sceptical Feminist* (Middlesex, Penguin, 1982), p. 113.

26 Margarete Sandelowski, "Fault Lines: Infertility and Imperilled Sisterhood," *Feminist Studies* 16, no. 1 (1990), pp. 33–51.

27 Ibid., p. 48.

28 Catherine McKinnon, "Feminism, Marxism, Method and the State: An Agenda for Theory," *Signs: A Journal of Women in Culture and Society* 7 (1982), p. 19.

29 Annette Baier, "What Do Women Want in a Moral Theory?" *Nous* 10 (1985), p. 5634.

30   Luce Irigaray, *This Sex which Is Not One,* ed. Catherine Porter and Carolyn Burke (Ithaca, Cornell University Press, 1985).

31   Sara Coakley, "Gender and Knowledge in Western Philosophy: The 'Man of Reason' and the Feminine 'Other' in Enlightenment and Romantic Thought," in Ann Carr and Elissabeth Schussler Fiorenza, eds., *The Special Nature of Women,* in Concilium, 1991/6. See also P. Lovibond, "Feminism and Postmodernism," *New Left Review* 178 (1989), pp. 5–28.

32   See, for example, Evelyn Fox Keller, *Reflections on Gender in Science* (New Haven, Yale University Press, 1985); Sandra Harding, "Is Gender a Variable in Conceptions of Rationality?" *Dialectica* 36 (1982), pp. 225–242.

33   Evelyn Fox Keller, "Feminism and Science," *Signs: A Journal of Women in Culture and Society* 7, no. 3 (1982), p. 593.

34   Keller, *Reflections on Gender and Science,* p. 78.

35   Sidney Callahan, "Does Gender Make a Difference in Moral Decision-making?" *Second Opinion: Health, Faith and Ethics* (Oct. 1991), p. 76.

36   On these terms see Max Charlesworth, *Life, Death, Genes and Ethics* (Sydney, ABC Books, 1989), ch. 1.

Making babies, making sense:

reproductive technologies, postmodernity,

and the ambiguities of feminism

Alison Caddick

In recent years some feminists have cast a more critical eye over the achieve-ments of second-wave feminism than the early flush of enthusiasm and sisterly solidarity once allowed. For example, Juliet Mitchell argues that the women's movement and feminist thought paid insufficient attention to the conditions of their second-wave emergence, which she identifies as a radical shift in the nature of capitalist productive relations. As a result, she says, second-wave feminism has most likely helped to install relations that will institute new divisions between women and men, and between different classes of women.[1] This is not to say that the revolutionary challenge of feminism to patriarchy and to capitalism is necessarily lessened, but rather that we must know the ground on which we stand if the reforms we advocate are to have the consequences we intend.

Julia Kristeva has also considered aspects of the emergence of second-wave feminism, long expressing a quite ambivalent attitude with respect to the move-ment's claims and intentions. Although she says little directly of the changing social circumstances of contemporary life, her framework is deeply sensitive to contemporary claims that liberation is attainable, and it points to the risk of cultural movements unreflectively establishing political hegemonies in their own right.[2] In not knowing the conditions of its new sociocultural commit-ments, understood psychoanalytically and linguistically by Kristeva, a move-ment might find itself tied to a form of existence and structures of power it had hoped to eschew.

The following review and critique of some feminist responses to the new re-productive technologies will also be guided by a proposition that casts second-wave feminism in a more critical light. Yet it will differ from the positions mentioned above in asserting that the new feminisms do not have a sufficient grasp of the emergent setting which has given rise both to the new technologies and to the feminist approaches now coexisting with them. I will call this setting variously the "information age" and "postmodernity" and pose as a central problem the emergence of a new form of the person. My contention is that the new feminisms generally lack insight into the constitutive conditions of their object—most broadly "woman" and her autonomy—and that this inadequacy carries over into specific considerations of the new reproductive technologies and related technoscientific practices.

Donna Haraway's work will later provide an entrée into these matters, for she makes clear aspects of a general social development, one of which second-wave feminism necessarily partakes. It becomes clear that feminism's many and varied approaches to destabilizing old orders of "the natural," in the form of raising as cultural questions what it is to be a woman or a man, are part of deeper strains in the culture. Everywhere these promote the transgression of what were once the society's categorical certainties. Given this, a certain complicity between second-wave feminism and a larger development of which it is not fully aware (and of which the biotechnological revolution is a key part) may be suggested. I mean this in the sense of how broadranging sociocultural transformations achieve a hold on people in multifarious and imperceptible ways, among the most opaque of these being the implicit experience and understanding of the body. To refer to Haraway's now famous figure, both second-wave feminism and the technosciences help to establish the "cyborg" as our late-twentieth-century ontology.[3] Not quite in Haraway's terms, the cyborg is a figure for an emerging "authenticity" of the experience of the body.

Nevertheless, this "complicity" affords feminism a highly ambiguous quality: that collusion with an emergent cultural form, yet also an uncanny prescience of a future that many among its number purvey with deep ambivalence. I will suggest that the sources of this ambivalence, and the instabilities it provokes, structure feminist writing, as they do—for a whole generation of women—a deeply personal experience of a confounding promise of liberation. In this light, some feminisms may be seen to contain, even if implicitly still, a challenge to the already lived, ambiguously embodied, form of the postmodern person. As I will argue, it remains for feminism to theorize the deep sources of the ambiguities that so many women, and many feminists, feel in our confrontation with the technosciences.

Radical feminism and reproductive technology
In commencing a review of feminist writing on the reproductive technologies, one can hardly ignore the groundbreaking work of Shulamith Firestone, whose

Dialectic of Sex[4] has had a lasting influence in the evolution of second-wave feminism. A key radical feminist text in the early women's movement, its very favorable representation of the reproductive technologies has been echoed many times over in feminist fiction where reproductive technologies have been the device by which worlds without gender have been constructed.[5] But where Firestone's text is drawn into feminist discussion today, it is often with embarrassment, and it is frequently employed as the self-evident counterpoint of subsequent developments in feminist thinking. Thus Firestone's utopia in which women's liberation is secured—most importantly as liberation from the reproductive body—has been challenged with various conceptions of woman's body as her "power" or "specificity," the problematic of the broad women's movement of that earlier period having undergone a decided shift. Rather than focusing on the "problem of women's bodies," a typically masculine formulation, attention has been turned to masculinity itself, and especially to its power of definition and "knowing" which, typically coded as neutral, may subvert even feminist theorizations.

This is the case then, with Firestone. Subsequent theoretical work more sensitive to philosophical issues and forms of argumentation readily helps us see the typical assumptions of the liberal-rational tradition structuring Firestone's argument. Specifically, the mind-body "normative dualism"[6] is asserted in the proposal that test-tube conception and gestation-tank technology will free women from a system of sex-class distinctions rooted in the biological body.[7] Rather than this pointing to a future free of the oppression of women, women as such will disappear altogether. Indeed, Firestone wishes "not just to eliminate male privilege but the sex distinction itself," the mission, which for her sharply distinguishes second-wave feminism from earlier feminist sentiment.[8] What Firestone does not see in this implicitly rationalist proposition is that it is a thoroughly gendered solution. Behind the apparent neutrality of the technological tool, employed in the name of liberation, stands the knowing subject, master of an essentially passive, or pacified, body. Indeed, in Firestone's scheme it can be said that "Mind" is materialized in the technologies as an intellectual dislocation of the body's mute and complex mode of being and knowing, just as it surely offers to sever aspects of the specificity of women's experience from their bodies. Firestone's position has been identified as a thoroughly androgynizing effort which in the implicit terms of the West's dualistic outlook means the triumph of the male term over and against an essentially absent "feminine"; of the "cogito" over the body.[9]

As a decided reaction against the kind of technological solution that Firestone proposes, there comes what is today by far the most prominent and politically vocal feminist approach to the reproductive technologies: the work of Gena Corea in the United States[10] and Robyn Rowland in Australia.[11] The international feminist journal, *Issues in Reproductive and Genetic Engineering*,[12] carries material of similar inclination, and the tenor of the Corea/Rowland critique finds even broader resonance in sections of what may still be considered the activist women's movement.[13] The Corea/Rowland type of approach stands outside the official structures of the public debate over the new reproductive technologies (which in Australia has been dubbed the "ethics debate"), in contrast to the pro-technology positions of liberal feminists which are prominent in the reports of ethics committees and bodies of review. But, at least in Australia, the Corea/Rowland view has been integral to the media's "balanced" reportage of the new reproductive technologies.[14] Far from the new reproductive technologies being neutral tools, for these writers they express a misogynist purpose that threatens to usurp women's remaining power of reproduction which has to this point avoided the colonizing efforts of patriarchal science.

Corea's and Rowland's work comes in what is now a long line of feminist research that has been dedicated to debunking as myth or ideology the liberal explanation of the intentions and achievements of modern medical science. On the one hand, far from the emancipatory promise of modern medicine having been fulfilled, there is disturbing evidence of women today suffering the consequences of a medical science that creates its own diseases and pathologies, a problem especially acute for women who are medicine's preeminent clients.[15] In the areas of fertility and early childhood, attention immediately turns to iatrogenic diseases, including the infertility that is so often the given reason for women seeking to join in vitro fertilization (IVF) programs.[16] On the other hand, more basic structural and cultural points are made as to the special relationship which women occupy in relation to medicine. Historically, it is discovered, "woman's body" emerges as the privileged object of modern medicine, just as a newly forming scientific practice defeats a realm of "women's knowledge" as superstition and witchcraft. The fate of the midwives and the "old women's tales" is counterposed to the rise of a scientific interest in obstetrics and gynecology; indeed, their construction as central disciplines of a patriarchal medicine.[17] The nexus of a form of control and a particular, and partial, epistemological outlook is thereby identified as at the heart of the modern medical enterprise.[18]

Corea and Rowland, while they make considerable play of the science-caused suffering of women, do not especially elaborate this longer term historical perspective. In this sense they take it for granted as part of the common store of feminist knowledge. Indeed, these authors are not concerned to delve into the assumptions of the narratives on which their work depends or to make much of their theoretical consequences. They intend primarily to make decisive interventions in the politics of reproduction as an urgently needed challenge to contemporary technoscientific developments. At this level their work has had a significant consciousness-raising effect. But I will argue that this has been at the cost ultimately of arguing a position not that different from Firestone's.

This is an effect of a certain "fundamentalism" in their approach which has seen them and their supporters calling for a complete halt to all IVF programs and related experimentation. This kind of criticism comes from various quarters within the women's movement. Rebecca Albury calls their attitude "absolutist" and sees them locked into the parameters of moral debate, so defined by the daily press.[19] Donna Haraway would consider an "anti science meta physics" to inform their work,[20] while Michelle Stanworth, introducing a recent British collection, finds both "unrealistic" and distinctly unhelpful to women the view that the new reproductive technologies are "an artificial invasion of the human body."[21] These writers would, it seems, see the problem as stemming from the kinds of categorical distinctions that the Corea/Rowland position implicitly makes. Paradoxically, it is at this level that, despite its antitechnology program, the logic of the Corea/Rowland position unites with that of Firestone's pro-technology stance.

Corea, for example, must be highly provocative to her critics when she describes her own work as "a scream of warning to other women."[22] This says a good deal about her depiction of the scientific setting and the method she employs. Indeed, the brief article, "The Egg-snatchers," from which this quotation comes, encapsulates aspects of the approach to science and technology of what some call the "culturalist feminists."[23] Here is the archetypical feminine, emotional outburst, an uncontrollable bodily eruption, as Corea witnesses with her very own and innocent eyes the scene of a crime too horrible for words. The innocent observer, concealing the feminist detective, she has filtered into a nightmare world of laboratory experimentation only to find herself the tortured object of a thoroughly distracted science. This science is in a world of its own, deaf to the cries of the laboratory animals it mutilates, so absorbed as to have no idea of the reasons for Corea's investigative enterprise. A science fiction horror story unfolds as a hidden reality in our midst *now*. And this is the real horror—that some alien logic is set on a course independent of and quite oblivious to a radically "other" sensibility for which the interloper's innocence and Corea's scream stand.

Corea's technique involves an effort to establish a distance for the feminine reader, thus throwing into contrast what are for her the distinctively masculine traits of a patriarchal, and misogynist, science. Where Corea feels closer to the laboratory animals, and thus to nature, than to the male researchers; where she views the magnified and enlarged photographs of parts of women's bodies as the strange artifacts of masculine abstraction/colonization; where she employs the metaphors of industrial capitalism to describe the consequences to reproduction of the new techniques,[24] the silent counterpoint of the "feminine" and natural is active, and the attitude of patriarchal conquest in science is confirmed.

Elsewhere Corea documents in detail developments in reproductive science and technology and clearly names them patriarchal and misogynist.[25] Robyn Rowland broadly concurs. Speaking of Brian Easlea's work on post-sixteenth century science she says:

> Though some benefits have accrued to people in general, science has mainly been used as a tool of suppression and violence, and his book traces the sadistic use of science against women. . . . The scientific ethic, as Overfield has commented, like capitalism and imperialism, is "based on exploitation, elimination of rivals, domination and oppression. . . . Sexist research has developed sexist technology and together they operate to 'move control of women's lives from women to men of the dominant group.'"[26]

Rowland also attempts to draw out the implications for ethical decision making of the kind of relationship between science and women which she and Corea highlight. Rowland is particularly perplexed by the feminist requirement of defending a "woman's right to control her own body" in the new circumstances of IVF technology and what appear to be its detrimental consequences for women. Yet how do you defend "choice" for women in the case of abortion and not in that of IVF?[27] Rowland answers this by strategically displacing "choice" with "control" as the relevant ethical issue.

Rowland then, like Corea, discerns a preeminently patriarchal logic of development in the medicalization and technologization of women's bodies. These, she says, "shape" women's lives, even creating some "needs"; certainly they work to confirm our "need" to mother in a "pro-natalist" patriarchal setting. But, as should be clear, these are *ideological* needs. They are related to an "ideology of motherhood,"[28] which is an effect of patriarchy, the maintenance of which is an implicit object of medical science. The nature of ideology, and thus "choice," in Rowland's scheme is revealed as an effect in consciousness, achieved through the external imposition of structures and values. Thus women's reproductive choice, an effect of women's "reproductive consciousness," is constructed and reinforced by policies of the state, through economic structures, and the "operation of a variety of rewards." At a psychological level: "People also parent because it draws social approval; it satisfies their need for a sense of continuity and immortality; [and] because they like children."[29] In turn, medical science works on the "myth of woman as mother" as a form of social control—"the social control of women through control over women's bodies and procreation."[30]

So wherever women are said to be choosing, the *circumstances* of their choice must be examined. Indeed, if circumstances are such that women are not actually gaining control over their own bodies—that basic requirement of women's autonomy—then the notion of choice itself may be a red herring. For Rowland, "choice" alone may be too individualistic a notion that ushers in reproductive scenarios of detriment to women as a group. So, "control" is elevated to the level of an absolute ethical goal, becoming the touchstone by which "real" as opposed to "ideological" choice may be credited.[31] As Rowland puts it: "When women claim the right to 'choose' reproductive technology, does this necessarily increase the control of women over that technology?"[32]

It also becomes clear here on just what basis maternity comes to be an apparent preoccupation of these writers. It is not that they want to privilege motherhood as a role for women.[33] The long-standing feminist goal to allow women to remain "childfree" should they so choose is, in these same terms, a basic commitment of Corea's and Rowland's position. Maternity is given prominence because the perceived technological assault on maternity today only heralds the end of what little choice, autonomy, and power women still have. Maternity has proved a crucial "bargaining chip" for women in their relations with men through the centuries. Following Mary O'Brien's thesis that men must attempt to usurp women's power because of their anxiety over paternity, motherhood may be seen as the "only power base from which [women] can negotiate the terms of their existence."[34] In some vague sense Adrienne Rich's thesis on the "experience" rather than the "institution" of motherhood is invoked to indicate that there must be something other than patriarchy involved in a desire to mother,[35] but what this "experience" is constituted in is not made clear. The primary lesson to be learned in this approach is that maternity is at the center of an essentially combative relationship between women and men, with women always fighting from behind.

In this view, "needs" are secondary effects of a power play; power is a possession. It follows that to gain autonomy, women have to hold onto power, to gain control. This does not necessarily mean that women will be better off if they control the technologies: these themselves may be "patriarchal." The point is to come to some agreement about what is in women's interests—what we might properly choose in order to gain control—and then go out and take hold of it. Though Rowland raises, and seems attracted to alternative notions of power than the "male" one—power conceived in the positive terms of the possession of a competence or of "energy," as opposed to that of competition and conquest—she is ultimately swayed by an argument for maintaining a politically engaged focus on patriarchal power relations.[36] On the one hand, women may come to know who they are and what they really want by elaborating their "experience"—in the face of the distorting influences of the "institution."[37] On the other, the combative edge of this radical feminism reigns, for masculinity seems always to be incorrigible.

Radical feminism's submerged body

Clearly the effort of Corea and Rowland to politicize woman's body, and reproduction in particular, upsets the claims of liberal-humanist medicine: the myth of scientific progress as the lessening of human suffering, the objectivity and neutrality of science and technological application. In one sense, too, technological determinism seems to be challenged for we are not simply to accept that culturally we lag behind science: indeed, we may fight it. Far from the technologies themselves unfolding some inner logic of their own, their unfolding is the expression of determinate interests, "science mirror[ing] the power relations in society."[38]

However, the *form* of this explanation is strikingly similar to the one it challenges. While the teleological unfolding of the liberal-humanist dream is apparently called into question, we have instead a dystopic teleology of "patriarchal" science embedded in an all-encompassing "truth" of men's quest to control women. It is the mirror image of the history it does not like. And while there appears to be a challenge to technodeterminism, the same gulf between technique and "humanity" that is assumed in notions of technique as mere tool and in that "magical" sense of technology as an alien force may be found in feminist accounts of this kind.[39] The latter is clear in Corea's depiction of the alien logic of a masculine science. In both Corea's and Rowland's work the notion of the patriarchy that lies behind a misogynist medicine is never scrutinized, but rather plays the same kind of mysterious role that technology often does. The former—the essentially instrumental understanding of technology— is evident in the notion of ideology as an effect in consciousness and that construal of power and needs I note above, both of which are completely consistent with the liberal-rationalist tradition. Neither ideology nor power here contains any sense of their role as constitutive, foreclosing the possibility of viewing the new technologies as bearers of a transformation of the body and person. On the one hand women are told that they are the dupes of patriarchal ideology; on the other we find that bodies, with their needs established in secondary relationship to their contexts, remain distinctly separated from the technologies that can only "intrude" into them.

Although we find here a reaction against the "technological fix," which apparently values and locates power in woman's body, a range of commitments common to both Firestone and the broader tradition in which her work can be situated comes to light. As has been pointed out elsewhere, the respective positions of early radical feminists like Firestone and later ones like Mary Daly, are reunited at a submerged level in a common project exactly with respect to the issue of "woman's body."[40] Where in Firestone women must forego their bodies and become more like men as an expressly androgynizing project, constructed on the dichotomizing categorical underpinnings of Western culture, in the so-called culturalist feminist case the intention to grant women a specificity is foiled because this position merely privileges the "silent" term of that structuring dichotomy, doing nothing to overthrow the basically "logocentric" orientation this entails.[41] Thus, in Corea's work where the category "woman" is set over against "man" as an unproblematized category, the effect is to accept a schema in which no real specificity is allowed. Similarly, while Rowland apparently challenges the liberal-rationalist discourse on rights and needs by exposing a structure of patriarchal power beneath their usage in the "ethics debate," her privileging of "control" as the arbiter of right depends on a conception of power that sees the instrumental separation of technology and the person, science and "humanity." In particular, where the "ideology of motherhood" thesis is employed, we find exactly that dichotomizing outlook that sets body against mind, rationality and will in a hierarchy over a passive, possession-like body.

In both these cases, then, I am suggesting that we do not find an adequate theory of the body. As the critique above suggests, the "body" is essentially taken for granted; whether in argument for or against the technologies, it remains the mere "body-appendage." And this, ironically—for Corea and Rowland, at least—entails the same assumption as the popular view that although the new technologies may in some sense be "revolutionary," essentially they change nothing. Love, common sense, the family—in the views of the scientists, liberal bioethicists, and a broad public—all stand as our guarantors of an unchanged "humanity." Our bodies, despite the changes they wreak and undergo, are the senseless appendages of those higher things that define what is good and proper.

Without an adequate theory of the relationships of bodies and persons to technologies, the intentions of feminists will be subverted. Clearly, the rosy liberal outlook with which many content themselves is quite foreign to both Firestone's position and that of Corea and Rowland at the level of their explicit statements. Firestone's Utopia bears little resemblance to the "mother's milk" view of a reproductively enlightened future. Corea and Rowland both predict the superoppression of women and nature when the scientists wrest the embryo from our bodies. In both cases, far-reaching consequences for our being and doing in the world are explicitly predicted, yet the methods employed do not in any way challenge the overarching framework of cultural coherence which the liberal rationalist view still, perhaps residually, offers. Though these writers seem to know that a general social shift is occurring, they do not have the conceptual wherewithal to represent it.

Intriguingly, Firestone's sense of a crucial break—her feeling for it, and her optimism about it—tend to link her more closely with the avowedly postmodern position of Donna Haraway, which I shall discuss presently. Corea and Rowland are more ambiguous. They deny any such break as they develop a picture of an increasingly entrenched patriarchal science. The message is that technoscientific reproduction only threatens us with more, albeit worse, of the same. But this picture is confused by Corea's dreadful "scream of warning." If we are to expect only more of the same, it would seem that this "knowledge" of the body is such as to cast technoscientific reproduction in the dimensions of that qualitative leap which grows of a quantitative development pushed to its extreme. For that scream of warning I believe, as with Firestone's optimism, "knows," even if these states of the body are not adequate to conceptualization, the revolutionary potentiality of technoscience for our everyday life. As I have suggested, this turns on an emergent body construct which technoscience lives off and practically facilitates—a metaphor for the new age and the lived embodiment of the social form it symbolizes. Haraway will convincingly, and positively, describe this as our late-twentieth-century "cyborg ontology."

Clearly, however, as I have indicated, there is no option but for Corea and Rowland's "cry of warning" to be a cry of nature, nor for Firestone's optimism to be anything but an unreflective expression of radical autonomy. Their explicit understandings and location of technoscience must fall short: it is the crucial break they sense but can only partially describe. Thus Corea/Rowland can only misrepresent the new techniques as like the mechanical processes of industrial capitalism, encapsulated in Corea's metaphor, the "mother machine." Thus Firestone, as I have already noted, depicts woman and her body as essentially outside history and may therefore readily see technoscience as the *only* possibility for women's deliverance from oppression.

Donna Haraway: cyborg life, cyborg consciousness

The old dominations of white capitalist patriarchy seem nostalgically innocent now: they normalize heterogeneity, e.g., into man and woman, white and black. "Advanced capitalism" and postmodernism release heterogeneity without a norm, and we are flattened, without subjectivity, which requires depth, even unfriendly and drowning depths. It is time to write the *Death of the Clinic*. The clinic's methods required bodies and works; we have texts and surfaces. Our dominations don't work by medicalisation and normalisation anymore; they work by networking, communications redesign, stress management. Normalisation gives way to automation, utter redundancy. Michel Foucault's *Birth of the Clinic, History of Sexuality* and *Discipline and Punish* name a form of power at its moment of implosion. The discourse of biopolitics gives way to technobabble, the language of the spliced substantive; no noun is left whole by the multi-nationals. These are their names, listed from one issue of *Science*: Tech-Knowledge, Genentech, Allergen, Hybritech. . . . If we are imprisoned by language, then escape from that prison house requires language poets, a kind of cultural restriction enzyme to cut the code; cyborg heteroglossia is one form of radical culture politics.[42]

Haraway catapults us into another world—another "reality" and another order of feminist theoretical sophistication. In her "Manifesto for Cyborgs" she throws down a challenge to feminists to see the circumstances of their discourse, especially that upon what may now properly be identified as "technoscience."[43] Unlike the feminist authors we have just been reviewing, Haraway sees in the circumstances of our lived reality a broad-reaching development which for her goes under the name of advanced capitalism. Its concomitant aesthetic-theoretical elaboration is, it would seem, "postmodernism." In this "period" the essences that lay submerged in the feminisms of Firestone and Corea/Rowland are simply untenable if one looks at the reality of scientific practice—and the realities it constructs. As a professed "socialist-feminist" (a socialist feminism that will not entertain "Marxism" but will "play" with "historical materialism"[44]), Haraway sees the information revolution as the material foundation of the new order and theorizes, or rather "plays" with, its consequences for women. This material reality is one that brings both new oppressions and new, radical, possibilities, suggesting also both the need for and possibility of deploying new methodologies for the feminist project.

This reality is figured for Haraway in her notion of the "cyborg"—a "cybernetic organism, a hybrid of machine and organism, a creature of social reality as well as a creature of fiction."[45] Here we have Haraway's "ironical" figure as a model for both a way of being as individuals and a way of politics, and what we are regardless of our choices inasmuch as the information revolution now casts us and the oppressions of our times in distinctively postmodern terms. Cyborgs are both the potentially radical grouping of the new international working class—the women, especially, of the new "homework economy"—whose identities are fractured, shifting, part of the great network of worldwide information, and those cultural radicals who actively embrace the cyborg form where it liberates us from the subject form of modernity, dispensing with all essentialisms, all myths of lineage and genesis.[46]

In its negative frame, the cyborg manifests as "technobabble"—that fracturing of the "substantive" according to the metaphor of information which seeks "a common language" without "noise." The information revolution, from which it seems there is no return, necessarily starts from the move common across the communications sciences and biology: *the translation of the world into a problem of coding.*[47] But feminists have the choice. They may counter the current power frame of the information revolution (in which "all resistance to instrumental control disappears and all heterogeneity can be submitted to disassembly, reassembly, investment, and exchange") by coding the cyborg self according to their ends. They must engage in a process of myth making or "cyborg writing" which "insists on noise and advocate[s] pollution."[48] The information revolution affords this possibility of "writing" in ways not previously available. Where bodies as such are contested entities, and with the flattening out of an earlier form of subjectivity, we are left with "surfaces," all the better and easier to "inscribe." This etched surface is ideal for achieving the kinds of radical cyborg "connections" that Haraway advocates. *Formally* the two cyborg possibilities that Haraway identifies do not differ: "The entire universe of objects that can be known scientifically must be formulated as problems in communications engineering (for the managers) or theories of the text (for those of us who would resist). Both are cyborg semiologies."[49] It is that the new form offers different choices, different outcomes within its more general embrace.

Haraway, then, offers a project for the body in the late-twentieth century. In contrast to other perspectives on "postindustrialism,"[50] here political and ideological battles will rage, with the body at their center, a continuing site of contestation and construction. Bodies are discursive or textual entities generally, the conventional products of particular historical circumstances—thus Haraway's partially positive reference to Foucault on the modern body. But it does seem that the body of postmodernity is more radically open to reinterpretation than any body before it. Once bodies come to be seen as information, as interactions between them and between their parts come to be seen as a matter of coding, or as texts, the relative opacity they enjoyed under modernity is circumvented. On one hand this has meant that the dominant technoscientific trajectory constructs in actuality, literally, not ironically as Haraway would wish it, the "cyborgs" which are part of what she names "the teleology of star wars." There is no relief here, only the deadly game of a science and technology which still believes in its humanist calling. On the other, if the information revolution can help us see the basis in "writing" of our relationship to the natural world and to machines, then we may choose our destiny without recourse to opposing, but formally the same, teleological frameworks for understanding science and technology. That is, feminism and other progressive movements need not seek for essentializing distinctions that would make them "different" from the totalizing pictures of patriarchal capitalism and humanist science. Liberated from *this*, "a cyborg world might be about lived social and bodily realities in which people are not afraid of their joint kinship with animals and machines, not afraid of permanently partial identities and contradictory standpoints."[51] Haraway thus suggests both a more fluid, reflective relationship to our cultural constructions, and in seeing through the authorizing moves of the sciences and technodeterminist ideologies, a new responsibility for our technological invention. This appears to include our own bodies as integrally formed within the given possibilities of the new sociocultural setting.

The contrast between the positions of Corea, Rowland, and Firestone and that of Haraway is, then, quite stark in several basic respects. A way around the essentialist categories dictated by the modern is found in the cyborg, which figures a radical transgression of the old boundaries, "heterogeneity without a norm" now achieved by the information technologies but also practiced radically via a postmodernist heteroglossia.[52] Haraway's own provocative transgression of the traditional boundaries of science writing and literature is a case in point. As well as the "deconstruction" of the masculine/feminine dichotomy being achieved, crucially the mind/body split inherent in the science or technology/"humanity" dichotomy is also transgressed. A constitutive role is afforded science[53] and technology, the body, "the natural," being conceived as real, lived "fictions"—things that we humans live and have "made up." Conversely, science and technology, indeed their epistemological foundations, are situated in the larger historical settings of sociocultural wholes—industrial capitalism/advanced capitalism.

Textuality and its limit

Clearly, Haraway's work offers a number of advances on that of the previous authors. She can conceptualize the new, identify a range of its key characteristics, point even to the contours of what I want to see as the new "body construct": the cyborg, a body of fictional limits, a surface on which new fictions may be written, the manifestation of the codes we manipulate, the body over which we may effect a new kind of "autonomous" control. These, I would suggest with Haraway, are aspects of the construction of bodies and a mode of the self that any discussion of the new reproductive technologies must take into account.

This is to endorse not just Haraway's reading of contemporary technoscientific productions, but at least some parts of her underlying epistemological orientation. The technosciences, and the new reproductive technologies within them, are not to be understood in the terms offered by the essentialist position discussed so far. Like the "natural" world science deals with generally, woman's body is no essential substance beyond the meaning frames of culture, but is differentially constituted exactly through practices like the scientific and technological. This is the case with maternity also; we may speak of "cyborg maternity"—maternity as an epistemological issue—just as we know it to be recast today as a cybernetic problem in biology. With respect to the latter, though women may make more or less intelligent and more or less informed choices about how they "use" technologies, we are talking about a more general transformation in the cultural setting within which choice is constructed and its meaning radically altered. To be concerned for women, for infertile women and IVF children as well, requires critical examination of how science and technology are part of an active construction of who we "know" ourselves to be. We must take absolutely seriously, and as a primary consideration, the proposition that science and technology exert, in the terms of a larger cultural setting, some kind of "productive" power over bodies and persons. With Haraway I agree that there is an integral tie between an "arbitrary" historical construction of the natural—the technoscientific mode of our practicing the natural—and an emergent mode of the person: we are living a reconstruction of our "ontology." This is our cyborg being, that common cultural form which nevertheless promises a proliferation of differences, the multiple possibilities that grow from a conception of the world as code.

So the cyborg is many things in Haraway's essay. It is the (constructed) reality that we must comprehend. Its credibility as a call to action, or ideological figure in that sense, depends in large part on the accuracy of her claim as to its reality: that of it being the embracing form of the life of subjects in late-capitalist society. Yet clearly the cyborg, which identifies a form of knowledge with our age, contains its simultaneous negation. It is like the Derridean notion of "erasure" by which we are to understand that all acts of naming, identifying, and closure are simultaneously erased.[54] This is the "let out," the escape to a diversity of meanings once we understand that access to the real is always mediated by the linguistic strategy used. And, admirably enough, Haraway's provocative notion of the cyborg and her postmodern linguistic "playfulness" leaves the reader in no doubt that in her case a deliberate rhetorical strategy has been deployed. It is out in the open that Haraway is positioning herself and the knowledge claims she is making with postmodernism, from the point of view of feminism. No disinterested inquiry here. Indeed, if we are to have knowledge of the real, then for Haraway such knowledge can only ever be the partial knowledge which the "situation" allows. Feminism is a form of "situated knowledge" which may guide scientific and other kinds of access to the real.

However, I wish to argue that in Haraway's work there is a level of a covert play for power which Haraway may not recognize, or on reflection wish to propagate. The problems of which I speak here I believe have their source in both methodological confusion and theoretical inadequacy. In particular, Haraway's use of the cyborg metaphor radically confuses the intellectual with the lived, in a sense I will make clear below. Haraway touches on this distinction in her own frank discussion of the problems constructionist and deconstructionist methodologies face: in one vein it is, ultimately, how to hang on to any sense of reality at all.

Now to counterpose the "intellectual" to the "lived" would be to provoke Haraway to the utmost, and this distinction might indeed appear to undo those areas of common agreement mentioned above. But I do not mean to drive a wedge between intellectual production and life: in a strong sense I am arguing that science and technology are key forces in informing the kind of people we are. In words not quite those of Haraway, embodying developments in culture more generally, science and technology are embroiled in the deep structures of social interaction and of the psychological make-up of the person. What I disagree with is Haraway's argument in her "Manifesto for Cyborgs" that the new forms of knowledge—whether the technocratic information order or the poetical heteroglossia which breaks out as a possibility under the same conditions of information—merely have a "surface" on which to work. I want to retain exactly the opposite proposition, that the body and person are "depth" formations, even given the recasting of the world as information, or the radical cyborg exhortations to "re-write" the body. Haraway's work reflects a conception of the body and person which, in its deep anxieties about essential being, can comprehend the world only in the image of the text. Far from there being an encounter with incommensurable "difference" or otherness as Haraway's notion of heterogeneity might have suggested, we learn nothing of embodied life or social being which is not vulnerable to the "textual." Yet it is exactly social practice and embodiment, as modalities of being rather than as particular "narrative," "sites," or "locations" from which particular meanings spring, that offer resistance—and arguably a structured one—to the making over of life in the image of the text. This is the project in which Haraway, together with the systems managers and reproductive technoscientists, is engaged, as the notions of both the "cyborg" and the "surface" attest.

Situated knowledge

These issues may be drawn out in the consideration of practical examples like the new reproductive technologies, even if it is not exactly clear what Haraway would say specifically about them. In one version of the cyborg, and at one level of reading it, there is nothing that would readily lead one to take up either an actively "pro" or "anti" stance on the reproductive technologies. If they were to be judged part of the "homogenizing" or technocratic strand of the information order, then cyborg feminists would fight them on nonessentialist grounds. But cyborg feminism could equally argue for them in some version of our being able to take control of our technological creations. In fact, the cyborg notion seems intended first and foremost to legitimize a feminist politics of science and technology: "(b)oth chimpanzees and artefacts have politics so why shouldn't we?";[55] the problem is establishing a field of knowledge as one equally of power. Indeed if we are to find more specific ethical guidance, beyond the broad need to politicize claims to knowledge and the concomitant principle of our taking responsibility for our constructed worlds, then we must turn to feminism itself, or those standpoints offered through women as bearers of "situated knowledges."

What loosely binds the various hyphenated "identities" of women (of black-lesbian women, of white-heterosexual women, etc.[56]) is the "situation" of their oppression; all the feminisms seek redress for the denial of women's autonomy, or recognition of what Haraway calls their "agency."[57] Feminism occupies a privileged moral ground in Haraway's cyborg essay.[58] But it is at this point that Haraway's reliance on metaphor, and the cyborg metaphor in particular, produces a circularity in her political argument, for this potential point of ethical justification—for the cyborg outlook—rests on an identification of feminism generally as the archetypal cyborg. Here, too, then, there can be no clear guidance on the practical question of the reproductive technologies or any other particular instance of the technosciences. All that can properly be said is that the ethical is the political: the ethical attitude is the politicizing and relativizing of that which we might otherwise believe to be a gift or curse of nature or God. At the same time, we must be drawn to the conclusion that if women's autonomy is figured by the cyborg—and second-wave feminism is historically, actually, and necessarily a cyborg phenomenon—then our feminist self-understanding and our ethical judgments are to be subordinated to the knowledge form(s) of the technoscientific era and their insistent social outcomes.

A further look at how Haraway handles the question of access to the real, and by implication ethical action, shows that the real message of Haraway's work, and the ethical imperative which is implied constantly in it, must be dealt with at the level of her epistemological assumptions and method. Now here Haraway seems to recognize complexities and problems, but the productive tension that she imagines to exist when she begins to talk about them, dissolves, I will argue, before what is an overriding logic in her position.

In the essay "Situated Knowledges" this supposed productive tension is presented as taking shape between the deconstructive on the one hand and the idea of embodiment and situated knowledges on the other. The former embraces the celebratory mode of the cyborg—that bold "clearing of a space" for the imaginative construction of an alternative reality; we know that anything is possible under the sign of the text. In feminism's fight with a masculine science, it is the possibility of arguing the "radical historical specificity, and so contestability" of scientific and technological constructions. "Situated knowledge," on the other hand, attempts to deal with the "multiple personality disorders" Haraway says are the result of just that kind of "epistemological electro-shock therapy,"[59] which is her deconstructive method. It is as if the "embodiment" and "situated knowledges" that feminism draws on is a counter to the irreality of deconstruction and the cybernetic hyper-real alike.[60] She seeks to bridge the perceived gap between "theory" and "experience" in an exhortation to develop a new way of seeing.[61]

Thus, one has the sense of two divergent approaches in contest. This is certainly the sense you get of the subject/writer who tries to hold divergent possibilities together. But perhaps this subjective struggle, which seems real enough, is but a lingering problem of the still not wholly reformed modern subject. For this apparent counterpositioning is, and could be, nothing of the kind. A felt dilemma is resolved at the level of the text, from the standpoint of the text. Where "embodiment" might have suggested some recognition of a mode of being heterogeneous and resistant to the reduction of the text, the logic of the information age holds sway. Thus bodies are *only* to be known as texts, and "situations" as the spatially arranged points of view at which particular textual phenomena emerge. The positional emphasis in "situated knowledge" confirms that we are dealing with the surface of the postmodern "map" which Jameson has exhorted us to put first as the necessary intellectual work of our time.[62] If there is something more to being embodied—which would pose as a primary issue the question of how to describe the nontextual modality out of which "textual" formations grow, then Haraway's method won't let us get to it. If there is something more to "the situation"—other dimensions of sociobodily engagement in the world—the textual and positional conception obscure them.[63] Likewise with her mention of the "unrepresentable" in a reference to the "many faces" of nature.[64] The epistemological answer to both her prob-

lem of a certain subjective (embodied) "dissonance" and to the question of "reality" and "nature" more generally for historians and philosophers of science,
lies in this rather "thin" conception of embodiment and the social "space."
What remains intractable to description and understanding can by degrees be
approached by letting "difference" speak—or, to put it in visual and spatial
terms from all perspectives. But such "perspectivalism" is "difference on one
plane,"[65] a spatial formulation. In Haraway's framework, it cannot be conceived
that there may be in embodiment and forms of social practice, and largely
closed off from the textual method, another order or register of difference—an
order or orders heterogeneous to the heterogeneity of one plane, according to
the one, cyborg principle.

Ironically, for I agree with Haraway's philosophical critique of positions like
Gena Corea's and Robyn Rowland's, it is with another order of difference that, I
suggest, such writers remain in touch. The fear of a certain disembodiment of
women at the hands of a radically abstracted technoscience is argued on essentialist foundations. It is consequently dismissed as anachronistic in these postmodern times. Yet there are ways of grappling with those aspects of embodiment that do not have to be explained thus. Thinkers like Julia Kristeva, for
instance, encounter and begin to give us ways of conceiving of the unrepresentable of embodied being and forms of social interaction, and yet may explain the
body and person as varied historical constructions.[66] Kristeva employs a double
framework of analysis that is sensitive to the socio-bodily modalities of touch
and smell and movement, to the emotional and its sources, the nature of which
must escape the fully textual approaches, and which as such illuminate the
mechanisms of cultural commitment to the forms of knowing and being that
live through us. Another approach is offered in the work of Geoff Sharp, which
generally informs this article.[67] Where Kristeva conceives of the heterogeneous
"orders" of our being in the sense of our emergence into culture—the "presym-
bolic" and the "symbolic"—Sharp's work raises the prospect of a more fully
social explanation of the body and person as living a complex interaction of
social forms. What the emergent order of the text/information cannot know,
and which in one sense we personally value when we go as far as IVF to have a
child, is a level or mode of desire and embodied being tied to a distinctive form
of social life.

An ethical guide also emerges here. If we are to live the pleasures of the
body—which also requires that we continue to live much of its pain—then it
may be that we will have to defend structural elements of a culture that the

postmodern now pronounces defunct. This is not at all to say we will find ourselves defending the maternal sacrifice, as figured in the Madonna and child, or what others so barrenly call the "pro-natalist" ideologies of the nuclear family. This is to refer to the ideological instance rather than to the formal characteristics of the sociocultural in any of its given historical elaborations. This points to the need for an investigation of the mechanisms of the forms of the social tie observable in different cultures and historical periods—the social forms of the construction of persons, and not the particular narratives of identification which now fill the pages of postmodern texts as invitations to pure difference.[68] The positions of Kristeva and Sharp strongly contradict the postmodern proposition that the body is a mere surface, providing tools for an examination of those realms of being taken for granted in everyday life, and thus especially vulnerable to the assumptions of the technoscientific age which actively eschew, if not actively begin to engineer away, their existence.

So, I would hold that far from the "cyborg" metaphor offering feminism a creative spur to political activity, it represents an impasse for thought and action. Haraway does not really come to grips, nor could her method allow her to, with the meaning and mode of life of the technoscientific era. Indeed, she steps in with the metaphor of the cyborg on discovering the "real" cyborg exactly at the point where our cyborg desires, those of the text, should be laid out for critical reflection. I want to use the cyborg metaphor not merely as a provocation, and not in Haraway's sense, but critically: as a figure for a general sociocultural form that must be grasped first as a social issue (not primarily an epistemological one) and critically set within these terms against its predecessors. I would suggest that far from the adoption of the cyborg encouraging an unlimited reflexivity, it closes off the possibility of asking the questions we most need to today.

Conclusion: post-cyborg?

In summary, I have proposed that the development of the new reproductive technologies carries through a more general transformation in the mode of the constitution of subjects. That is, in line with much recent social theory—but hardly applied in the specific case of the reproductive technologies—I take the view that persons are constituted as such in distinctive and variable ways according to the sociocultural context of their personal formation. In particular, some theorists of and commentators on postmodernity help us begin to illuminate the distinctive self of postmodern society, pointing to the contemporary science-technology nexus as crucially implicated in the new subject form. For the purposes of this essay—which has sought to critique a range of feminist responses to the technologies—I drew on the work of Donna Haraway. The contrasting positions of Shulamith Firestone, of Gena Corea and Robyn Rowland, are the familiar terrain of contemporary feminist reproductive politics. All, however, fail to grapple with the emergent social reality partly carried in, certainly figured by, the new reproductive technologies; and none has a sufficiently developed theoretical apparatus with which to account for the relationship between technoscience and the person, especially the newly reproductively "autonomous" woman. These approaches can all be found to be deficient when a critique of their philosophical presuppositions and methodological orientations is undertaken.

So, Haraway's work—which suggests the notion of the "cyborg" as our distinctive mode of being and experience of the body in the information age—moves beyond the modernist assumptions of the previous writers. Hers is the provocative challenge to feminism in general to come to terms with a new reality, which demands radically new tools of analysis and elaboration. Ultimately, Haraway's position, as I have argued, carries deep problems for the feminist response to the technosciences. While she correctly identifies aspects of our new mode of being and helps to convincingly overturn the radical feminist and realist positions, she far too readily accepts the cyborg nature of our emergent desires. I have indicated how, though specific ethical guides are not to be found in Haraway's work, at the level of her methodological commitments, a definite logic of engagement in the world emerges. Here I suggest that although Haraway arrives at her conclusions by somewhat more acceptable means than Firestone, they both end in a celebration of the arrival of the information age. Finally, I point to some other approaches that indicate how feminism might overcome the impasse which for me Haraway's work represents.

Running through this article are assumptions that only really come to the forefront in these suggestions for alternative research directions. They are part of a preoccupation with the emergence of forms of the self and their lived embodiment. While Haraway must put forth an entirely textual account of the body, I wish to explore contrary forms of being, and to suggest that these coexist in our personal formation. Knowing better what these other orders of (socially constituted) "difference" or modes of (social) being are, we have a better basis for asking what the new reproductive technologies mean—for better posing questions about a widespread sense that "something" is put under threat by the new technologies. With the benefit of this kind of point of view, we may also begin to place second-wave feminism, and the contests within it in the form of the many feminisms, rather more adequately than is typically the case. Not only do different intellectual traditions and novel intellectual developments compete across groups of feminist thinkers and differently "situated (feminist) identities," a contest, or at least a confrontation, between different forms of knowing and being may be said to occur within and as the body of our ambiguous passage into postmodernity. In this light, some aspects of theoretically "outmoded" feminism may still offer insights into a more "human" alternative to the cyborg. At any rate, both Haraway's work, and the critique I attempt here I hope will help better situate feminism's quest for women's autonomy.

Notes

1 Juliet Mitchell, "Reflections on Twenty Years of Feminism," in Juliet Mitchell and Ann Oakley, *What Is Feminism?* (Oxford, Basil Blackwell, 1986).

2 Julia Kristeva, "Women's Time," in Toril Moi, ed., *The Kristeva Reader* (Oxford, Basil Blackwell, 1986).

3 Donna Haraway, "A Manifesto for Cyborgs: Science, Technology, and Socialist Feminism in the 1980s," *Australian Feminist Studies* 4 (autumn 1987): 1–42.

4 Shulamith Firestone, *The Dialectic of Sex: The Case for Feminist Revolution* (New York, Bantam, 1972).

5 For example, Marge Piercy, *Woman on the Edge of Time* (New York, Fawcett Crest, 1976), and see Susan H. Lees, "Motherhood in Feminist Utopias," in Ruby Rohrlich and Elaine Hoffman Baruch, eds., *Women in Search of Utopias* (New York, Schocken, 1984).

6 Jean Bethke Elshtain, "Against Androgyny," *Telos* 47 (spring 1981): 5–21.

7 For an outline of Firestone's notion of the body as a biological entity, see Alison Caddick, "Feminism and the Body," *Arena* 74 1986: 60–88.

8 Firestone, *Dialectic of Sex*, p. 11.

9 On Firestone in particular, see Elshtain, "Against Androgyny." But this is a point made more generally by many poststructuralist theoretical feminists, including Luce Irigaray, *The Sex which Is Not One* (Ithaca, N.Y., Cornell University Press, 1985); Iris Marion Young, "Impartiality and the Civic Public, Some Implications of Feminist Critiques of Moral and Political Theory," in Seyla Benhabib and Drucilla Cornell, eds., *Feminism as Critique* (Cambridge, Polity, 1987); or Drucilla Cornell and Adam Thurshwell, "Feminism, Negativity, Intersubjectivity," in the same collection; or Elizabeth Grosz, *Sexual Subversions, Three French Feminisms* (North Sydney, Allen and Unwin, 1989); Grosz's "Glossary," pp. xiv–xxiii, outlines key terms here.

10 Gena Corea, *The Mother Machine: Reproductive Technologies from Artificial Insemination to Artificial Wombs* (New York, Harper and Row, 1986); Gena Corea, Renata Duelli Klein, et al., *Man-made Women: How New Reproductive Technologies Affect Women* (London, Hutchison,

1985), and various articles, including 'How the New Reproductive Technologies Could Be Used to Apply the Brothel Model of Social Control over Women," *Women's Studies International Forum* 8, no 4: 299–305.

11   Robyn Rowland has written many articles, both for the popular media and scholarly audiences, and many conference papers. For example: *Woman Herself, A Transdisciplinary Perspective on Women's Identity* (Melbourne, Oxford University Press, 1988); "Reproductive Technologies: The Final Solution to the Woman Question?", in Rita Arditti, Renate Duelli Klein, and Shelley Minded, eds., *Test-tube Women, What Future for Motherhood?* (London, Pandora Press, 1984); "Choice or Control? Women and Our Relationship to the New Reproductive Technologies," paper delivered to the Conference on Liberation or Loss? Women Act on the New Reproductive Technologies, Canberra, May 1986; "A Child at Any Cost?", *Connexions, an International Women's Quarterly* 32 (1990).

12   *Issues in Reproductive and Genetic Engineering: A Journal of International Feminist Analysis,* (New York, Pergamon Press) ed., Robyn Rowland (Australia) and Gena Corea (United States).

13   For example, the American magazine *Connexions* (see issue no. 32, 1990), but also evident as a relatively popular view held on the technologies among feminists as local conferences, on feminist radio programs, and in other discussions.

14   Robyn Rowland and Renate Klein are the two feminists in this "camp" who almost exclusively have been called on by the Australian media to comment on developments and represent the feminist point of view locally, e.g. the Melbourne *Age* over several years, the popular Peter Couchman forum series on ABC TV.

15   For example, morbidity and mortality rates related to medical advice given on the bottle feeding of children in the third world, as well as concerns about the side effects of the oral contraceptive pill, Depo-Provera, and intrauterine devices.

16   For example Hilary Rose, in her diagnosis of the new reproductive technologies, "Victorian Values in the Test-Tube: The Politics of Reproductive Science and Technology," in Michelle Stanworth, *Reproductive Technologies, Gender, Motherhood, and Medicine* (Cambridge, Polity, 1987). The identification of iatrogenic infertility encourages her to a "socioecological" approach, p. 172; Rowland, *Woman Herself,* pp. 135, 164.

17   Barbara Ehrenreich and Deidre English, *For Her Own Good: One Hundred and Fifty Years of Experts' Advice to Women* (New York, Doubleday, 1979); Brian Easlea, *Science and Sexual Oppression: Patriarchy's Confrontation with Woman and Nature* (London, Weidenfield and Nicolson, 1981); also Adrienne Rich, *Of Woman Born: Motherhood as Experience and Institution* (London, Virago, 1982).

18   On the epistemology/power/gender nexus in modernity, see Carolyn Merchant, *The Death of Nature: Women, Ecology and the Scientific Revolution* (New York, Harper and Row, 1980); Ehreinrich and English, *For Her Own Good*; and E. A. Grosz and Marie de Lapervanche, "Feminism and Science," in *Crossing Boundaries* (North Sydney, Allen and Unwin, 1988). On women's newly medicalized role in the "preservation of children," see Jacques Donzelot, *The Policing of Families* (New York, Random House, 1979); Michel Foucault, "Hysterization of Women's Bodies," *The History of Sexuality: An Introduction* (Harmondsworth, Penguin, 1987). For the epistemological issues proper, see Sandra Harding, *The Science Question in Feminism* (Ithaca, Cornell University Press, 1986).

19 Rebecca M. Albury, " 'Babies Kept on Ice': Aspects of the Australian Press Coverage on IVF," *Australian Feminist Studies* 4 (autumn 1987): 63–64.

20 Haraway, "Manifesto for Cyborgs," p. 37.

21 Stanworth quoting Klein in "The Deconstruction of Motherhood," *Reproductive Technologies,* p. 35.

22 Corea, "The Egg Snatchers," in *Test-tube Women,* p. 48.

23 For example, Juliette Zipper and Selma Sevenhuijsen, "Surrogacy: Feminist Notions of Motherhood Reconsidered," in Stanworth, *Reproductive Technologies.*

24 The references to mechanical process and industrial capitalism are throughout *The Mother Machine,* and in many of the articles in *Test-tube Women* the same kinds of metaphors are to be found, for example, "Designer Genes: A View from the Factory" and "Inside the Surrogate Industry."

25 *Mother Machine.*

26 Rowland, *Woman Herself,* p. 45.

27 Rowland, "Choice or Control?", p. 2. In fact, one finds that by posing this question, neither Corea nor Rowland is in practice absolutely opposed to technological intervention in reproduction or to science generally. Apart from arguing for abortifacient technologies, they also concur with feminist arguments for a transformation of science, in part through the encouragement of greater numbers of women scientists who, they assume, will do science differently. Their "fundamentalism" is not so much a matter of their statements as to do with a level of unacknowledged assumption, which makes for logical contradictions vis-à-vis their broad intention to challenge the patriarchal character of reproductive science.

28 Ibid., pp. 6–7.

29 Rowland, *Woman Herself,* pp. 6–7.

30 Ibid., pp. 163–164.

31 Rowland, "Choice or Control?", pp. 6–7.

32 Ibid., p. 4.

33 Stanworth, "The Deconstruction of Motherhood," holds the view that these feminists overvalue motherhood.

34 Rowland, "Choice or Control?"

35 Rich, *Of Woman Born.*

36 Rowland, *Woman Herself,* pp. 153–154.

37 See Rowland's chapter in *Woman Herself,* "Culture and Self-creation through Writing," pp. 66–87.

38 Arditti et al., "Introduction," p. 4.

39 The mysterious force of technology is often commented on in the literature on technology, related to perceptions of the inevitable unfolding of some supposed internal logic. See Stephen Hill, *The Tragedy of Technology, Human Liberation versus Domination in the Late Twentieth Century* (London, Pluto Press, 1988, chapter 1).

40 Elshtain, "Against Androgyny"; Caddick, "Feminism and the Body."

41 Haraway, "Manifesto for Cyborgs," p. 6 for example, but for elaborations of the theme of logocentric thought, see Irigaray, *This Sex,* and Kristeva, "Women's Time."

42 Haraway, "Manifesto for Cyborgs," p. 6 (footnote).

43   "Technoscience" refers to the interpenetration of science and technology in the historically novel sense that advances in one are basically dependent on the other: theoretical science informs technological development directly and scientific discovery is dependent on the powers of the new science-based technologies.

44   Haraway, "Manifesto for Cyborgs," e.g. pp. 12–14.

45   Ibid., p. 1.

46   See also Haraway, "In the Beginning Was the Word: The Genesis of Biological Theory," *Signs* (spring 1981): 469–481.

47   Haraway, "Manifesto for Cyborgs," p. 19 (her emphasis).

48   Ibid., p. 31.

49   Ibid., p. 17.

50   For example, Francis Fukuyama, "The End of History," *Fortune* (January 1990).

51   Haraway, "Manifesto for Cyborgs," p. 8.

52   On postmodernist heteroglossia, see Brian McHale, *Postmodernist Fiction* (New York, Methuen, 1987).

53   See Haraway, "Manifesto for Cyborgs," pp. 18–19, for example.

54   See Gayatri Chackravorty Spivak's "Translator's Preface" to Jacques Derrida, *Of Grammatology* (Baltimore and London, Johns Hopkins University Press, 1976), pp. xiv–xviii.

55   Haraway, "Manifesto for Cyborgs," p. 5.

56   Ibid., p. 8, "Fractured Identities."

57   Haraway, "Introduction" to *Simians, Cyborgs and Women, Reinventing Nature* (London, Free Association Books, 1991), p. 3.

58   Haraway, "Manifesto for Cyborgs."

59   Haraway, "Situated Knowledges," in *Simians, Cyborgs and Women*, p. 186.

60   Ibid., p. 184.

61   Ibid., in the section "The Persistence of Vision," pp. 188–191.

62   Frederic Jameson, "Postmodernism, or the Cultural Logic of Late Capitalism," *New Left Review* 146 (1984): pp. 53–92.

63   The modern notion of the "situation" provides a useful contrast to Haraway's idea of "situatedness." According to Sharp, a defining feature of the contemporary period is the disintegration of the situation as the primary setting of the constitution of the self and integration of persons into society. It is exactly the kinds of network formations Haraway identifies and the image technologies that transgress national and ethnic boundaries, as well as those of the modern institutions, which break up the situation. "Situation" refers to a specific "density" of relations between persons and things, a less abstracted engagement of the body in the world, and a particular notion of social "causality." The "density" of which I speak implies a depth of intuitive meaning and value, which is a casualty in the information society where the "network" and the "interface" are the emergent dominant mode of social connection. See Sharp, in "Keywords: the Network," *Arena Magazine,* no. 10, April–May 1994, pp. 46–47, and Caddick, in "Keywords: Subject Positions," *Arena Magazine,* no. 12, August–September 1994, pp. 39–40. Haraway is worried about "boundless difference," but her challenge to this with respect to relationships in the world is conceived in the depthless imagery/language of the information mode itself: the "task of making partial, real connection," ("Manifesto for Cyborgs," p. 51).

64 Haraway, "Introduction," *Simians, Cyborgs and Women*, p. 3.

65 This refers to Geoff Sharp's work on "constitutive abstraction." See his "Constitutive Abstraction and Social Practice," especially the sections "The Abstraction of the Cultural Frame: The Emergence of Autonomy" and "The Ideology of Autonomy and Cultural Contradiction," *Arena* 70 (1985): 68–76.

66 Kristeva, *Revolution in Poetic Language*; see Moi for excerpts, pp. 89–136.

67 Sharp, "Constitutive Abstraction and Social Practice."

68 For example, the three volumes of *Fragments for a History of the Human Body* (New York, Zone Books, 1989).

Bodies and subjects:

medical ethics and feminism

Philipa Rothfield

> His face was a simple graft grown on collagen and shark-cartilage polysac-
> charides, smooth and hideous. It was one of the nastiest pieces of elective
> surgery Case had ever seen. When Angelo smiled revealing the razor-sharp
> canines of some large animal, Case was actually relieved. Toothbud trans-
> plants. He's seen that before.[1]

Medical ethics, especially bioethics, is a shifting terrain. Medical and reproductive technologies threaten the stability of categories once regarded as biological
absolutes.

> "You can't let the little pricks generation-gap you," Molly said.[2]

Perhaps the field is a response to these instabilities, an attempt to fill "the gap".
For example, the technological denaturalization of the category "reproduction"
raises questions about the plasticity of the body and sexual difference, invoking
deeply ethical and political concerns. Similarly, genetic engineering poses problems regarding the boundaries and character of human being.

> Molly had gone back to the loft hours ago, the Flatline's construct in her
> green bag, and Case had been drinking steadily ever since. It was disturb-
> ing to think of the Flatline as a construct, a hardwired ROM cassette rep-
> licating a dead man's skills, obsessions, knee-jerk responses.[3]

It is not as if one could determine the *objects* of the field, i.e., genetics, without
at the same time *positioning* oneself and the field in relation to ethical questions.
Or could one? Gibson's novel, *Neuromancer,* from which the above quotations
are taken, is a science-fiction story that imagines a future structured by incred-
ible developments in computers, genetics, cybernetics, robotics, and artificial
intelligence. It is set in a totally reactionary, violent social milieu. Although a
great adventure in cowboy cyber-punk, no thought is given at any stage to the

ethical implications of what people (or things) do to each other, or how society is run. A great deal of human being has become artificially rendered: the body comes to be thought of as meat, dead flesh, the most crude of substances when compared to the pure, white, crystalline structure of computer reality, the quasi-hallucinogenic site of the "real" adventure:

> Cyberspace. A consensual hallucination experienced daily by billions of legitimate operators. . . . A graphic representation of data abstracted from the banks of every computer in the human system.[4]

In contrast, the simulated experience of another person's corporeal sensations is considered distasteful, it being "basically a meat toy," representing a "gratuitous multiplication of flesh input."[5] The disavowal of the body here—its replacement by machine or silicon chip—allows the technological fantasy of disembodiment, abstracted hallucination, and the dismemberment of ethical matters in regard to the body.

Diprose, in contrast, writes of the *primacy of embodiment* (the fact that we are bodily selves) for any sense of biomedical ethics.[6] She discusses the body and ethics in a way which blocks the imaginary exclusions (or corporeal self-hatred) so prevalent in Gibson's novel. A notion of embodied subjectivity, such as Diprose uses, contradicts the *disembodied universalism* that is so often invoked in ethical discussions. Feminists have criticized the abstracted disembodiment of the humanist subject (the abstract individual), positing sexual difference as a paradigm of difference and embodied specificity.[7]

My aim in this article is to approach medical ethics by exploring that upon which it depends, namely an understanding of the body. This represents a shift away from the body *as object* toward an attempt to develop a sense (or senses) of embodiment and its multiple relations with medical ethics. When one begins to explore embodiment, ramifications can be felt vis-à-vis the once disembodied subject of knowledge—here perhaps the ethical subject, the practicing medico, or the speculative theorist/philosopher—as well as in relation to its field of objects. In a paper this size, I do not intend to synthesize a complete reconstitution of the field; rather, I shall select a few themes and issues in relation to the body and embodiment.

However it is arrived at, a particular sense (or senses) of what the body is will have implications as to how medical ethics understands the embodied subject of medical practice (the patient). A medical ethics which adopted a particular view would be affected not merely in terms of *the body as object* but also with respect to *the knowing ethical subject*. A note on terminology: by subject I mean person. In this immediate context, there is a subject of medical practice—the person being treated—and what is referred to as the knowing subject, that which occupies the (implicit) position of knower in a field of knowledge.

I first question whether there is/should be *one* sense of embodiment. Scientific and medical knowledge is generally articulated in a fashion that suggests a singular bodily knowledge, one that underlies all human beings. This bodily knowledge is totalizing. It represents one (universal) sense of embodiment, albeit one that acknowledges differences between actual (particular) bodies. But it does not acknowledge, recognize as valid, or accept the existence of differences between distinct *forms* of bodily knowledge. *Gray's Anatomy*, for example, has sections on the differences between the male and female pelvis, and between the organs of "generation."[8] Otherwise, the one body is represented in terms of a number of interlocking systems: blood-vascular, musculo-skeletal, lymphatic, nervous. The text presupposes that it makes no difference where or how a body is embodied as regards the generality and validity of the work, which is a treatise on anatomy. Its framework exhibits a universal indifference toward the particular body, concentrating instead on the minutiae of differences within the one generalized, subdivided body. In general, the medical case history, so graphically depicted in medical magazines, serves to refine or rebut medical knowledge of the body. Particular bodies instantiate or contradict universal claims about human bodies. Their function within medicine is to enhance the (cumulative) growth of knowledge. It is not the case that medical claims about bodies are regarded as *themselves* particular (and therefore limited) bodies of knowledge. This is a matter which is repressed in the formulation of medical knowledge.

As I write, I realize that other forms of medicine—holistic, traditional, Chinese, indigenous—are beginning to be recognized by what I characterize as a univocal and totalizing form of knowledge: Western, conventional medicine. However, where "unorthodox" medicine (a potential aberration) is considered, its recognition is granted subject to medical understanding and scientific method. Hence, unconventional medicine is tested according to the methods of conventional medicine and science. Its "truth" depends on successful scientific trials. It is not treated as a parallel or possibly incommensurable field of practice and knowledge, nor as a field whose insights may surpass those of medical science, nor as a partial perspective among others including that of medical science, but it figures within an epistemological (knowledge) hierarchy that governs the projected field.

The following example illustrates the ways in which conventional medicine deals with the unorthodox. In 1992, the *Australian Doctor Weekly* published a series of articles on alternative medicine. One article, on natural therapy, began with the views of a naturopath who is the chairperson of a statewide natural therapy association, a Mr. Tasker, who stated that he was "not concerned that natural therapies cannot be explained in conventional terms."[9] The first section of the article dealing with naturopathy ended with the claim that conventional medicine is now recognizing the value of "dietary management" and has always taken the patient's well-being to be an important aspect of general practice. In other words, either medicine appropriates the insights of naturopathy or it already knew that which naturopathy knows. The next section, on homeopathy was entitled, "Troubles." The "trouble" with homeopathy, unlike naturopathy, is that its theoretical and practical basis has elements which are, in the quoted words of a clinical pharmacologist, "*totally contrary* to the basic principles of pharmacology." This is more difficult than the case of naturopathy, for anything that contradicts medical views "must" be treated with suspicion. After talking of double-blind tests, dose-response curves, and what conventional medicine does believe and accept, Associate Professor Shenfield ended on a positive note, speaking of the areas of overlap between alternative and conventional medicine: where homeopathy's claims are common with those of conventional medicine, there is less of a problem; the trouble arises where there is contradiction. Mr. Tasker, on the other hand, said that naturopaths did not claim to have all the answers. He was quite prepared to see his own field as incomplete and complemented by orthodox medicine. In an accompanying article on registration requirements (i.e., institutional credentials), we are informed that accredited courses for naturopathy "are said to be at the standard of an undergraduate degree in science." Note the equivalence relation is drawn between a science degree and the naturopathy qualification, as if science is the yardstick for any form of recognition.

Subjects and theories

I question whether there is one and only one sense of embodiment (whether that given by Western medicine or any other account) partly on the basis on feminist and French theories of difference. Once the body is refracted (and multiplied) through notions of difference, the body and bodies of knowledge are thought in terms of their specificity, partiality, and multiplicities. My other reason for questioning whether there is one sense of embodiment is that, later in this piece, I try to develop a practice-based notion of embodiment which incorporates a subjective sense of one's body and the ways in which the subject moves, both conscious and nonconscious. This approach leaves room for many forms of embodiment, which is why I criticize what I see to be the unitary understanding so often expressed within anatomical works. What may be shared (and therefore common within a culture if not universal) is the discursive context within which we form our sense and modes of bodily being.

Much of the work on the body which is informed by French poststructuralist thought regards knowledge as *discursively produced*—that is, issuing from a particular sociohistorical context, its representations, forms of knowledge, and institutions and social practices, all of which go to position and produce subjects of knowledge. This is to question the idea that knowledge somehow captures, reflects, and represents the way the world is.[10] The epistemological suspicion which this entails is extended to medical knowledge by looking at the kinds of frameworks it presupposes, its historical and social settings, and its social practices.[11] Rather than knowledge being separate from its object, the two (subject and object of knowledge) are regarded as mutually complicit: Western medicine, its practices and frameworks of understanding, are bound up with that which is known according to these fields.

Feminists associated with this (French) tradition look at the way in which knowledge and theory is articulated in relation to sexual difference.[12] They deny the neutral epistemological subject, analyzing neutrality in terms of a covert masculinity:

> From a feminist standpoint, the inadequacy of the theoretical model of classical rationality is that it is oblivious to sexual difference in that it mistakes the masculine bias for a universal mode of enunciation. The sexual neutrality it professes conceals a fundamental and unspoken phallocentrism.[13]

If feminism has done anything, it has drawn aside the curtain on the scene of (theoretical) representation, *marking the place* from which it ensues, the gender and interests it serves. In other words, feminists have drawn attention to authorship, the place both real and implicit in the text which has been male-dominated for so long. A great deal of effort has been expended in feminism to expose masculine bias and to contest its purported neutrality.

These forms of feminism theorize sexual difference as a crucial marker, not merely of the objects of thought, but also of the subject of thought, what I here call *the knowing ethical subject*. I have been working in feminism so long that I take it for granted that my work expresses a feminist subject position—that is, that the implied author of this text takes a feminist perspective, presupposes and speaks to a body of feminist work. At times, that perspective will expressly concern itself with questions of the female body, sexuality, and sexual difference. More generally, it manifests as a concern over difference and an acceptance that the positions taken here are not universal, disembodied, or disinterested. This recognition of *positioning* has connections with other forms of political theory that also acknowledge and pursue work over difference. For feminism, it is inter alia difference from an unacknowledged masculinity that purports universality in the form of gender neutrality. For some postcolonial work, it is difference from Western perspectives whose ethnocentrism coupled with colonial privilege blinds it to its impositions upon the non-West. One difference is not the same as another, and each region of analysis may well invite criticism from other regions as to its own blind spots.[14]

There are political and historical bases for sexism, racism, and ethnocentrism that both mask a covert masculinity, white dominance, or Western ethnocentrism, while allowing for the expression and imposition of an apparent neutrality/universality. Often those who have developed critiques of this universality expressly declare themselves as not universal and neutral, for example, a black critique of racism. Also, women of color have criticized the unacknowledged racism and white dominance of what purports to be a universal feminism. Two illustrations:

> Have you read the grievances some of our sisters express on being among the few women chosen for a "Special Third World Women's Issue" or being the only Third World Woman at readings, workshops or meetings? . . . [We] continue in most cases to be treated as "temporary sojourners", even though we may spend a lifetime by their side pleading a common cause.[15]

And for Aihwa Ong:

> The papers as a whole tell us more about Marxist feminist thinking about the capitalist world system than about the experience of women and men in the industrialising situation. . . . By portraying women in non-Western societies as identical and interchangeable, and more exploited than women in dominant capitalist societies, liberal and socialist feminists alike encode a belief in their own superiority.[16]

Finally, postcolonial theorists are working on the ways in which colonialism has exported and imposed Western modes of thought and domination on the non-West. For example, Edward Said's work, *Orientalism,* shows the history of Western forms of knowledge of the Orient and the ways those in the Middle East have been subjected to these forms of knowledge. Said documents and traces the formation of learned societies in Europe in the eighteenth and nineteenth centuries, their academic institutionalization, and the colonial relations that enabled and enhanced these processes.[17] In Said's account, "Orientalism" says more about the European subject of this form of knowledge, and colonial power relations, than about its supposed object, "the Oriental."

In each of these illustrations, power differences have enabled one interest to espouse and assert its neutrality or objectivity and required another to assert its difference as a means of criticizing the neutrality of the dominant interest. Dipesh Chakrabarty has written of his own project in postcolonial Indian history as requiring a literacy in what he calls European history, as well as in Indian.[18] He says that part of his work involves "parochializing" history, showing the extent to which it is European—that is, its specificity rather than its purported generality.

I mention these areas of thought because they each question whether knowledge is able to represent an all-inclusive, neutral, disembodied perspective.[19] The embodiment of perspective as regards knowledge, its positioning, will have implications for any purported universality of medical knowledge. I raise then a double sense of embodiment—of self as well as of perspective. By self I mean that the human subject is an embodied creature. The abstract individual of Enlightenment thought which represents the subject of reason can be thought of as a mind whose body has been abstracted away and associated with reason's Other(s), whether emotion, imagination, body, or woman. The embodied individual is an attempt to rethink such a disembodied mode of abstraction. The other sense of embodiment, that of perspective, is a reference to the previous discussion regarding knowledge: that knowledge always arises from a complex of circumstances, practices, related forms of knowledge, and institutional loci. It is not a panoramic view of the world but is always partial, provisional, and located.

Bodies and subjectivity

Western medicine would seem to apply a singular form of knowledge to the human body, an apparently reasonable assumption given the worldwide applicability of drugs. Penicillin, for example, can be found to be effective throughout the world equally (even though many third world people cannot afford it). The suggestion is that global usage implies a singular bodily form. And yet the relation could go the other way around, such that what we have instead is the spread of multinational drug companies as part of global capitalism. In other words, global imposition can masquerade as some kind of universal givenness; economics masquerades as logic. Either way around, there are other forms of therapy, healing, and health that give very different accounts of the human body and human being from that of Western medicine. Are these accounts to be *subsumed* under the Western paradigm? Or are they *incommensurable* with Western concepts of the body? If they are incommensurable, is one account to be rejected? Consider Chinese medicine, acupuncture, and shiatsu which have a different mapping of the body, elaborated in terms of energies, elements, and meridians. Some professionals utilize both forms of medicine in their practice, for example, using acupuncture as anesthetic for surgical intervention, or treating a bad back with acupuncture, infra-red heat, and anti-inflammatory drugs. For this practice to be "coherent," is it necessary to reduce these two models to one?

An answer to this question depends not only on a sense of what coherence requires but also on one's view of the body: whether it has a singular or multiple character, whether all humans share the same kind of body, or whether there are numerous bodies depending on a variety of circumstance, history, and location. Moira Gatens writes of there being at least two bodies, the male and the female, but also of the imaginary body, the lived body, and the situated body.[20] These terms presume an account of bodily specificity—bodily difference, rather than bodily sameness. By difference is suggested a sense of specificity that discourages the assertion of a total system of bodily coding such as anatomy might be taken to represent but rather focuses on the ways in which actual bodies are specifically produced, and the differences between these forms of production. Elizabeth Grosz has written that "Feminists have increasingly recognised that there is no monolithic category, 'the body'. There are only *particular kinds of bodies*.[21] She writes of the "socio-political production of determinate historical bodies."[22] If there are many kinds of bodies, multiple lived forms of corporeality, is medical ethics able and willing to deal with this diversity? An answer to this will partly depend on whether medical ethics is conceived of as a unitary and universal project or a number of diverse ethical spheres. It also depends on how medical practice is conceived—that is, whether it is seen as an umbrella category to whose understanding all bodily forms are subject or as one practice among others.

Intervention

Medicine is sometimes described as a practice of intervention. This could be taken to suggest that there is something there, already well formed (i.e., autonomous) that is being treated. It is also possible to argue that *the form of intervention is bound up with its own object,* in which case the self-conception and conceptual framework of medicine, its character, is intimate with a certain kind of body and a certain notion of illness, intervention, and health. To illustrate: if the doctor is perceived by all as the expert, the one with the knowledge of the patient's body, this may pacify the patient's body as well as posit no bodily knowledge on the part of the patient. The doctor is knowledgeable and responsible, the patient is subjected to the expertise of the Other. The hierarchy of the hospital and clinic may testify to the doctor's knowing what the patient and the lay community does not. The structure, timing, and costing of the session, the provision of prescribed drug information to the doctor and not the patient—these do not just support this kind of "ignorance" but they help produce it. A group called Healthsharing Women has been set up in Melbourne to make information available to women on matters of health to break down this kind of approach. I have heard a similar account of the chiropractor's intervention, which consists of "fixing" the patient by manipulating the person's spine. If the person is sent off without learning any more about how his/her body works, why the problem arose, no knowledge of the patient's body is produced within the patient. It may also be the case that the chiropractor doesn't know, either— that the spine is just "out," and the approach is to manipulate it back into shape. But if the work itself involves manipulation on the part of the practitioner, the cure residing in the therapist, the patient is similarly ignored as the epistemological subject in regard to his/her own body. A lot of this depends on both the intention and the character of the intervention. Some doctors spend the time explaining things to their patients. Also, some alternative therapists, whose form of therapy might claim to work on the subject's understanding, could jut apply their framework, whether naturopathic or homeopathic without engendering any growth of understanding in the subject. However, some techniques such as Alexander and Feldenkrais, are predicated on bodily awareness by the *subject* and require a kinaesthetic dialogue involving the subject's understanding of his/her own body *in order to proceed.* Feldenkrais writes: "In my lessons the student learns to listen to the instruction while he is actually carrying out an exercise and to make the necessary adjustments without stopping the movement itself. *In this way he learns to act while he thinks and to think while he acts.*"[23]

I want to examine these two ways of characterizing intervention: intervention on the given versus intervention as production. The latter concept of production may be seen to act in two directions, that is, producing both the body acted upon and the intervening therapist. I shall begin by elaborating these differences of approach in relation to two views of reality.

The objective world versus the world as produced

The extent to which ethical issues intrude on what might be regarded as conceptually independent matters (matters concerning the objects of the field) depends on the kind of outlook adopted. If intervention is a form of production of both body and practitioner, then it may well be an ethical matter *what* form of production is involved. If, on the other hand, intervention is an act upon a given body, ethical matters arise in relation to the *act of intervention*, not the *process of production*. I want to explore this difference in terms of two theoretical outlooks: (1) The first approach emphasizes objectivity, and the *givenness and independence of reality*. Let us call this an *objectivist* approach.[24] (2) The second approach theorizes the *discursive production of reality*, knowledge, and the world. Let us call this a *productivist* approach.

These two attitudes are not peculiar to medical ethics but loosely cluster around two philosophical traditions. It is possible to associate the first approach with Anglo-American philosophy, which is generally informed by a realist tradition, referential theories of meaning, and an epistemic valorization of ontology and metaphysics. The second can be associated with French structuralism and poststructuralism, which variously emphasize the systemic or discursive production of meaning, subjects, and reality. It is sometimes traced to the philosophical skepticism and nihilism of Nietzsche and Heidegger on the one hand, and a hybrid antirealism based on the work of the linguist Saussure on the other. It could be pointed out that neither approach adequately reflects the complexity and diversity of either associated tradition. This is certainly the case. I characterize these two metaphysical tendencies in order to explore the body, its givenness, its agency, and the sense in which it is culturally constituted. I am also interested in the *substance* of the body and its relation to culture, discourse, and epistemology. So, to some extent, these two theoretical approaches are imaginary, "hyperreal" terms in Chakrabarty's sense.[25] They do not have exact referents but are idealized heuristic constructions. I use these two terms to elaborate an ontology and epistemology of the body.

In the first, objectivist approach, it is possible to know the world independently of the account in which knowledge is articulated, who it is who knows, and the relevant and related field(s) of knowledge (e.g., medicine, philosophy, and feminism). Knowledge is the *transparent* means by which reality is understood. The aim of knowledge is to give a true, justified account of the world. The forms of justification may vary from field to field, but the clarity and neutrality of the knowledge relation holds. It is neutral with respect to the subjects and objects of knowledge, as well as the field of the particular subject matter.

In the second, productivist approach, knowledge is not neutral with respect to the above-mentioned factors. The world cannot be accessed independently of language, culture, and discourse, and these factors are epistemologically opaque. Those who occupy the position of knower may well lend (if not impose) their own character to the knowledge created. Put conversely, the position of the knowing subject is bound up with a given form of knowledge. Here knowledge plays an active even a *constitutive* part in generating the nature of that which is known. The world is knowledge or theory dependent: knowledge participates in the construction of reality. In the productivist approach, the being of the world is not understood as merely objectively given. The world is understood as a complexity that cannot be reduced to some neutrally given set of objects or state of affairs. For both accounts, there is a reality, there are positivities, but in the one case, it is there to be understood, and in the latter, that which is understood has been produced and therefore may be further investigated. These forms of production cluster around both the known object and the epistemological relation between subject and object. They affect the known object, the knowing subject, and the relation between the two.

The productivist approach represents a kind of skepticism toward the idea that reality can be known qua reality as it is in itself.[26] The world can only ever be understood via linguistic or discursive relations which themselves have much to say about its character. Even people (subjects) are caught within, and produced by, this combination of representation, practice, and institution, called *discourse*. The elements of an objectivist epistemology—reality, the knower, and the field of knowledge—are here conceived to be part of social, semantic, and cultural processes rather than outside (or epistemologically prior to) them. "Objectivity" is thus always articulated within a complex network of signifying relations and practices.

There are two points to be made about reality with respect to the productivist approach. First, there *is* a sense of reality. It is not reduced to consciousness, perception, or intersubjectivity. The productivist approach does not exclude materiality. The point is rather that we can never know that materiality independently of its discursive determination. To borrow a locution from Ros Diprose, the real is inextricably caught within its representation(s). The inextricable melding of matter and its discursive representation consist of sociohistorically located "events." Their forms are particular and historical so that theorists such as Foucault make it their business to elucidate the ways in which this has occurred. His work is always historically focused, showing that the givenness of reality is a historical production. Notice the following way in which Foucault discusses science, the systematic knowledge of reality:

> It is a question of what *governs* statements, and the way in which they *govern* each other so as to constitute a set of propositions which are scientifically acceptable and hence capable of being verified or falsified by scientific procedures. In short, there is a problem of the regime, the politics of the scientific statement. At this level, it's not so much a matter of knowing what external power imposes itself on science, as of what effects of power circulate among scientific statements, what constitutes, as it were, their internal regime of power, and how and why at certain moments that regime undergoes a global modification.[27]

Foucault is concerned with what kind of reality a particular discursive regime makes possible—its "truth-effects" as he puts it—rather than the true as such. His work is often concerned with historical shifts in knowledge (the discursive regime), and that which is both utilized and brought into being in effecting such a shift. Notice, once a "reality" is made "possible" via these changes in regime, discourse, and technology, it is also real *within* that sphere's dominion. He does not expose the production of reality as a false process that conceals an underlying veracity that he wants to indicate. Foucault's aim is to show the ways and means by which that reality came about and to contest the notion that reality is passively, objectively "there," awaiting discovery. To that extent, his work stands as an argument against objectivism. For example, in *Discipline and Punish,* Foucault traces the shift in punishment from the public spectacle of torture and execution to the individualizing processes of incarceration and reform. Along with the development of the modern prison came many techniques and forms of knowledge, indeed a "whole set of assessing, diagnostic, prognostic, normative judgements concerning the criminal have become lodged in the framework of penal judgement." Foucault's work on these multiple forms of science, and technology which participate in the exercise of the European criminal justice system is at the same time said to be "a correlative history of the modern soul" and a new power to judge. For Foucault, a new individual is produced by these various procedures, techniques, knowledges and practices, what he calls "the modern soul". That production arises from a process of "epistemologico-juridical formation" wherein the human sciences and penal law are jointly produced.[28]

All of these processes, effects of power as he would put it, are real. But the individual, the modern soul, is a (real) effect of these processes, not an autonomous (prior) object upon which these processes operate. Thus, it is both real and produced. Foucault uses the word "positive" to indicate that these complex processes are not merely repressive—that is, they do not just act on the individual but *effect* one.[29] This is at the heart of the productivist orientation.

From the production of consciousness to the production of the body

The production of subjectivity (personhood) is an intrinsic part of the productivist approach. In some versions of the approach, consciousness is seen to be the product of social processes, whether via interpellation in Althusser's antihumanist Marxism[30] or social construction according to some forms of feminism and socialisation theory.[31] In both cases, the human subject, the self is produced.

Very briefly, in Althusser's version, ideology is the means by which we come to be individual selves. The role of ideology within all societies is to produce subjects suitable to the processes of the social formation (society). Part of the content of that subjectivity is the belief that we are individual subjects. It is a form of subjectivity that is produced. We come to think of ourselves as individual subjects because we are constantly addressed as subjects within social practice. We "recognize" ourselves as such in these forms of address to the point of thinking ourselves constitutive (or humanist) subjects, and we attribute our consciousness to an identity we regard as self-produced, as our own.

Within feminism, it is masculinity and femininity, our gender identity, that is said to be socially produced. The sex/gender distinction separated two forms of identity: sex, which is anatomical, and gender, which is associated with social roles. The sex/gender distinction was employed within feminism to allow for a separation of that which is anatomically given (sex) from that which is socially constructed (gender). The *givenness of the anatomical body* was contrasted with the *social plasticity of the constructed gender identity,* and the latter was valorized as the sphere of social change.

Identification of the subject with consciousness has been criticized by Foucault (with respect to Althusserian Marxism) and Moira Gatens (with respect to feminism) as part of a joint rejection of Cartesian Dualism. *The result has been to reintroduce the body as a central term for any account of subjectivity.* Moira Gatens has criticized the sex/gender distinction as a separation that ascribes all the processes of social construction to the mind, and not to the body, which is seen as unchanging, anatomical, and given.[32] She attributes the separation to Cartesian Dualism which she rejects, arguing that the production of the body is part of the socially produced self and is not outside social determination. Similarly, Foucault has criticized Althusser for developing a theory of the subject within Marxism via ideology's focus on consciousness and not the body.[33] Both these criticisms aim to introduce the body into the sphere of "social construction" (subject-production) as a means to counter its tendency to be consciousness-centered, and as a way of acknowledging the materiality of these processes and of the subject him/herself. The result is that the body comes to be understood *through* discourse, not outside of it. So the body which is being introduced can be described as a *discursive body,* not as an anatomical given.

It is really in virtue of both feminism and Foucault's work that the body has become important within what I call the productivist paradigm. It represents a convergence of the theory of the subject (personhood) with a productivist approach wherein the subject is no longer identified with consciousness but also incorporates the body. The crucial point is that the body here is seen to be *produced* rather than given, and that production implies a certain materiality out of which a subject is formed. The term *embodied subjectivity* has been used to imply a rejection of Cartesian Dualism and the introjection of the body into the theory of subjectivity.

Within the context of this discussion, I think that something needs to be said regarding whether the body is to be regarded as having a universal (singular) structure or can only be spoken of in particular senses. We have seen how two divergent philosophical orientations accompany each possibility. The objectivist approach underlies the universalism of medical knowledge, whereas the productivist approach is able to engender a multiple set of (possibly incommensurable) knowledges. Productivism is able to underlie multiple knowledges because it is not committed to the existence of a reality "out there" as the object of knowledge. Were that to be so, it would not be possible to consider incommensurable knowledges, for either a state of affairs obtains or it does not. If knowledge is "flavored" by the knowing process and the subject of knowledge, it is possible to conceive of many kinds of knowledge which are the result of various discursive processes. The many forms of reality arise through discursive *folies à deux* between subject and object of knowledge. For productivism, the existence of multiple corporeal forms or modes would be tied to the discursive social processes within which bodies appear. The latter would point to a social, semantic, and institutional basis as being in part responsible for any multiple modes of bodily being.

Objectivism, on the other hand, lends itself to the view that there is one kind of bodily being (embodiment)—whether that being is topographically male or female—and thus, there is one system of bodily knowledge. Were there to be many kinds of bodies or forms of embodiment according to objectivism, it would have to be on the basis that multiple corporeal modalities were in existence. In other words, the emphasis of objectivism would be on the existence of diverse bodily forms and not on a multiplicity of ways in which they were known. Similarly, if objectivism is to conceive of multiple systems of bodily knowledge, these systems would have to be interlocking and compatible—e.g., the muscular, skeletal, and nervous systems; they might also include naturopathy and its "compatibility" with orthodox medicine.

In the next section, I make some attempt to reconcile an element usually associated with objectivism (substance) with a productivist account of inscription. This occurs in relation to changing the self/body and that which both enables and constrains bodily being, its substance and form. Since I do not posit bodily matter as separable from that which produces the embodied subject, this is not an objectivist viewpoint. It is much more aligned with an elaboration of productivism, but it is coupled with an insistence on bodily matter. How is this insistence to be spelled out?

Critical reflections

The discursive approach toward the body, or the production of bodies, is often articulated in terms of *bodily inscription,* in which the body is socially and culturally inscribed by various discourses, and this is interiorized to produce a sense of subjectivity.[34] Let me begin by raising some problems I have in regard to the discursive bodily approach or ways of rendering the productivist paradigm. They have to do with a tendency to *avoid* the body, insofar as it is represented by the body's anatomy and physiology, and a more general evasion of the corporeality and materiality of the body.

Rejection of the anatomical body is a consequence of the desire to avoid essentialism. Essentialism within feminism, and in this context, has been associated with the view that there are essential differences between men and women, and these are grounded in biology. Here essentialism is linked with biologism. Any attempt to ground sexual difference in biology was thought to affirm an immutable, objective basis for masculinity and femininity. First, Moira Gatens has written: "Theorists of sexual difference do not take as their object of study *the physical body, the anatomical body, the neutral, dead body,* but the body as lived, the animate body—the situated body."[35] Notice that here the physical body is inert—it's dead meat.[36] Part of Gatens' reasoning, I take it, is to introduce lived, alive, situated, and sexually differentiated bodies. But the price of these bodies entering would seem to be the cost of the physical, dead, anatomical body.

Vicki Kirby provides a second set of examples in the context of a discussion of corporeality, feminism, and essentialism.[37] She analyzes a number of readings of Luce Irigaray, a French feminist of the body and sexual difference, whereby Irigaray has been read in such a way that the body is regarded as discursive, imaginary, rhetorical, or poetic; anything but "real" flesh and blood. Kirby refers to a paper that was read aloud on the work of Irigaray, where the speaker argued that Irigaray was not essentialist by saying that she was not talking about the body in "this" sense, and pinched herself.[38] I find it interesting in this latter case to see the *presence* of the body equated with some notion of the anatomical or biological body (to be avoided at all costs) as if it is not also a social and cultural body, and therefore a discursive one at the same time. So strong is the desire to reject the anatomical body that its physical presence is excluded from the ambit of discussion.

The difficulties Kirby depicts arise also because of a reluctance to make a referential gesture toward the body. The work of Derrida is sometimes taken to proscribe all forms of reference. Kirby denies this. She writes that Derrida's work *problematizes* reference but does not exclude it altogether.[39] In any case, there are good political reasons for asserting an ontology of bodies and their differences, including sexual differences. Rosi Braidotti writes:

> The starting point, however, remains the political will to assert the speci-ficity of the lived, female bodily experience, the refusal to disembody sexual difference into a new allegedly postmodern anti-essentialist subject, and the will to re-connect the whole debate on difference to the bodily existence and experience of women.[40]

Surely a refusal to disembody must carry with it some recognition of concrete existence? Kirby's criticism of feminist writers such as Gallop, Whitford, and Burke concerns their tendency to discuss the body in a textual rather than physical fashion. Perhaps the danger of biologism outweighs the desire to acknowledge the physical, concrete body. "Gallop is not alone in excluding biology from consideration. There seems to be an almost consensual agreement amongst Irigaray's most sophisticated defenders that a limit must be deter-mined with regard to the notion of materiality, textuality or anatomy in Iri-garay's texts."[41]

I think another reason to be textual rather than physical is that bodies are theorized in a textual manner, the stuff of theorization. The physicality of bodies is once removed from the text, even though all authors are embodied, all communicative interchanges full of interacting bodies, and all acts of reading performed by embodied subjects.

Elspeth Probyn writes of the difficulties associated with "mentioning" the body in academic contexts. She wants to keep the *body in speech* apart from the *body in reality,* arguing that the former tends to slip into the latter, and that the body in speech is thereby expected to speak some truth, the truth of reality. The danger as Probyn sees it is that a realist epistemology creeps in as soon as reference is made to actual bodies, the "body at hand."[42]

Pointing the finger

In the following, I want to explore what is thought to be ostended (pointed to) in referential gestures. Although theoretical discussions of the body are quali-fied and nuanced, reference is somehow conceived of as a brute gesture. It is not at all clear what ostension does. The philosopher Wittgenstein writes of osten-sive definition as a language game of its own, open to interpretation in all cases, dependent on circumstances and on those to whom it is made.[43] It is not a simple matter of pointing, for one still has to say *what* is being pointed to.

If the anatomical body were to be indicated, what would that mean? Does one point to the corpse of anatomy in referring to the body "in reality"? In *Birth of the Clinic,* Foucault traces the period in which it became permissible to cut up dead bodies for medical investigation and autopsy, a practice that ultimately lead to the creation of pathological anatomy. Foucault describes the physician Bichat's analysis of the volume of the body via a conception of tissular space (bodily tissue). The dissection of bodies enabled the development of this knowledge, its excavated surfaces allowing the mapping of a three-dimensional corporeal space. Death provided a great insight into diseases of the living:

> But Bichat did more than free medicine of its fear of death. He integrated that death into a technical and conceptual totality in which it assumed its specific characteristics and its fundamental value as experience. So much so that the great break in the history of Western medicine dates precisely from the moment clinical experience became the anatomo-clinical gaze.[44]

Bichat's *Anatomie generale* was first published in 1801, his *Anatomie pathologique* in 1825. The dissecting gaze of anatomy is still manifest today. *Gray's Anatomy,* a current classic of the English language, first published in 1858, includes a cellular and tissue analysis. Its sections each have directions for dissecting particular regions and parts of the body. This is partly for teaching purposes— medical students are provided with dead bodies for dissection.[45] This perspective also structures the way in which anatomy is understood as a form of knowledge. The knowledge which constitutes the anatomical gaze is based on the work of dissection—a morbid and pathological (sick) anatomy.

Knowing how to cut up bodies is undoubtedly a useful medical skill. However, there is no reason to accept that anatomy must be defined by the gaze and logic of dissection. Let us consider Andrea Olsen's text, *Bodystories: A Guide to Experiential Anatomy:*

> Our skeleton is alive. The 206 bones in the human body are living tissue. . . . Bodies change throughout our lifetime. . . . They are affected by evolutionary and genetic heritage, but also by proprioceptive stimulation, balance of body weights through the skeleton, diet, exercise, trauma, illnesses and injuries, emotional experiences, and life patterns of work and play.[46]

Olsen's work on experiential anatomy attempts to facilitate bodily understanding via text and practice. The narrative on bones, for example, is accompanied by practical sections such as "Articulating the Bones" and "Moving from Bone." The text does not say what the subject should feel. It simply directs the subject through a number of exploratory movements or thoughts. This sense of the anatomical body is alive. Its epistemology is tied to the subject's awareness. Its understanding of the body is in part constituted by the subject's own perceptions as they arise in the work of the practical sections. Even though little time is spent on cultural and sexual differences, beyond their acknowledgment, the experiential element of the practical work allows for variations of response, perception, and feeling.

I mention Olsen's work not because it is *the* answer to the problems of traditional anatomy; it merely represents a practical, movement-oriented approach to anatomy which constitutes it as an understanding of the structures and forms of *lived bodily experience.* Olsen's anatomical body is not dead, although it does relate to classical anatomical knowledge: for there is talk of bones, a photo of a skeleton. However, these are interspersed with artistic drawings, calligraphy, photos, representations from a variety of cultures, and abstracted images and works. No particular priority is given to the orthodox representations of anatomy.

If anatomy could never acknowledge the discursive element of embodiment, it would be severely limited; if anatomy begins with the living present body, however, there is no need to assume that such a body is located outside discourse or that anatomy requires *one* kind of body.

Olsen's approach to anatomy represents an interest in the present body; it does not substitute the dead body for lived experience, and it need not deny the determinations and productivity of discursive inscription. Its starting point is merely the presence of the body. The present body can be thought of as the figure/site of many determinations—discursive, semantic, and signifying. Certainly, it need not be thought of as pure biological matter, a belief that seems to underlie the avoidance of corporeal presence.

What, then, is being ostended (in the reference to actual bodies), and what kind of gesture of ostension is being made? To point to the corpse of anatomy requires the hand (and gaze) of the dissecting physician as well as pointing to the body as a corpse. To point to Olsen's experiential anatomical body is something altogether different, for this is not a pointing from the outside (a visual gesture) but more a form of listening, one in which it is not assumed what is being listened to.

The intention to indicate the present body, the body at hand, could be any or none of these things. The realist expectations that are supposed to accompany any reference to the body arise because an empirical object is picked out—that is, the body is located as a knowable object of the real world. This is to assume that, like G. E. Moore's "A Defence of Common Sense," to say here is a body is to imply that we are entitled to take its existence and nature for granted; that I know this is a body and roughly what it is.[47] However, as Wittgenstein has argued, it is not all that clear what form of knowledge common sense implies. If I claim to know "here is my hand," what does this mean?:

> #59 "I know" is here a *logical* insight. Only realism can't be proved by means of it.
> #83 The *truth* of certain empirical propositions belongs to our frame of reference.[48]

Just as Foucault makes it very clear that the gaze—its epistemological framework, institutions, and technologies—determine what can be seen, the gesture of pointing has its own choreography, setting, and multiple agendas of interpretation that also affect what is ultimately regarded as "the object" of ostension. Even the potentially intransigent corpse of anatomy could be resuscitated in different ways.

The presence of the body is not necessarily the "truth" of the matter. Being "here" does not yet reveal what being consists of nor bring with it any epistemological guarantees.[49] The substance of the body, its apparent solidity, should not be mistaken for epistemological transparency or analytic fixity. The body has volume, but one that is constantly moving, changing from day to day, moment to moment. It is open to multiple internal experiences; outside interpretations; conscious, imaginary, and unconscious representations; and it is penetrated by discursive forms of determination. It is clearly an overdetermined site, one whose strands cannot be simply unraveled.

Thinking substance

I chose the two extremes of objectivism and productivism because they are forms of opposite on the matter of bodily substance. For objectivism, bodies are given—*found objects*—whereas for productivism, bodies are produced: *made objects*.[50] The latter's object status is neither simple nor simply given. I shall describe three senses of the production of bodies:

1. *The forms of production are pure representations.* The tendency here is to reduce the body to a form of textuality. This textuality was the subject of Kirby's concern in relation to feminist approaches to the body in Luce Iri-

garay's work and regarding a more general avoidance of essentialism in feminism. Because the body's matter is identified with an extracultural body, it is *excluded* and textual representation becomes the sole focus. This is to ignore the materiality of the body beyond that of its textual representations. The body is a form of textual immanence because ontological reference is not on.

2. *The body is a conjunction of matter plus representation.* This acknowledges the material substance of the body, and it claims that we never have access to that substance independent of its discursive inscription. But this approach slips into a Kantian division between matter as the thing-in-itself and representation as a discursive veneer or imprint upon that basic matter. Its problem is that it suggests the existence of a fundamental substance, a noumenal matter, which exists outside of and prior to discourse, culture, and society. It differs from objectivism on epistemological grounds in that we never have access to the fundamental substance of bodies, but, like objectivism, there is a suggestion that corporeal givenness exists independently of and prior to subjective, epistemological, and discursive influence. I think a version of this approach lies behind the fear of bodily presence and ontological reference. The thought is that reference is an attempt to pick out this fundamental substance—indeed, that "real" bodies are tainted by the blood of referential matter.

3. *Matter and its representations are inextricably bound together.* It is not possible to speak of one or have access to one independently of the other. There is no noumenal matter. I aim for a version of this third approach.

The differences between 2 and 3 are subtle. It is difficult not to allow 3 to slide into a form of 2—namely, to suggest there is an underlying form of pure, bodily substance. Reference to an inextricable melding of matter and representation makes no realist epistemological assertion, however, for that which is referred to is already part of representational networks. If this is the stuff of which presence is constructed, then ostension need not be avoided.

Another way of indicating the inextricability of substance and its forms of representation is via the notion of inscription and its surfaces, for neither surfaces nor their inscriptions are pre-given (constituted independently of one another). Any aspect, region, or process of the body can function as a surface of inscription. It may be part of the body's interior (under the skin) or its exterior. The point of using the term *surface* is to indicate that it is liable to inscription.

Thus, internal aspects of the body are also inscribed. One can speak of anatomical, physiological aspects of the body as already penetrated by inscriptive processes. Indeed, Foucault's work on dissection and anatomy in *Birth of the Clinic* traces quite clearly the way in which dissection both carved bodily surfaces, created a certain kind of gaze, and constructed a means of analyzing the corporeal dimensions of the body. The crystallization of that analysis as knowledge became anatomy, a system of representation which penetrated the body according to a dissecting logic.

Perhaps we need to explore what is meant by surface. There is a tendency to assume surface implies exteriority. This need not be so. Surface can be thought of as a dimension or a process which becomes rendered in some way or other. It is a surface *of* something or *for* a process (here, of inscription). What it is not is a depth, with some internal essence. In other words, that which is a surface is not pre-given. Surfaces are corporeal, material constructs. They are the material interfaces of inscription.

In general, I am sympathetic to accounts that focus on the discursive production of bodies. I do not believe that the body is an objective given, whose nature is independent of the sorts of discourses through which it is understood. In that sense, I do not regard inscription as something that can be easily sloughed off, but neither do I think the body is an utterly malleable, plastic entity. Bodies are not sponges, computers, blank sheets of paper, or empty vessels. They are living flesh, with blood, bones, organs, and energies. Even if bodies are inscribed, and forms of bodily pleasure are produced, there is the (material) stuff that *interacts* with these processes. This is why I use the terms *corporeal constructs* and *material interface* to indicate that there is a materiality of the body which participates in the inscription process. Materiality is not thought of as an objective pre-given reality. Its reality only arises through the inscriptive process. My concern now is to spell out that interaction between substance and inscription.

Elizabeth Grosz comes the closest to acknowledging the "stuff" of the body and its inscription: "The metaphorics of *body-writing* poses the body, its epidermic surface, muscular-skeletal frame, ligaments, joints, blood vessels and internal organs, as *corporeal surfaces* on which engraving inscription or "graffiti" are etched."[51] She later gestures to the raw materials and basic units of inscription. She thereby acknowledges that biological, anatomical, physiological, and neurophysiological processes may provide a "universal or quasi-universal" "bedrock," a bodily materiality, marked by inscription. So, for Grosz, biology and anatomy interact with inscription. Perhaps, she writes, the body is less like a blank page than a "copperplate to be etched":[52] *the character of inscription has to be intimate with that which is being inscribed.* Like the technologies and materials of artistic inscription, the viscosity of the paint, the surface and qualities of the paper will have a great effect on the form as well as the result of inscription. Video art is another example: the sort of work created is reflective of the equipment, the colors available, the technology utilized, and the videotape itself. Thus, surfaces are not pre-given, and neither are forms of inscription.

Inscription and its surfaces

We are now at a complex moment in the argument in that the interaction between inscription and that which is inscribed resists reduction (in either direction). Objectivism is rejected in that it reduces the discursive to a contingent veneer. And equally, inscription is not the whole story, for there is that which is inscribed which similarly cannot be bracketed off. Version 2 of productivism is rejected for its separation of substance which is thought to *preexist* discursive inscription. In an interview, Foucault mentioned that in an early draft of *The History of Sexuality,* vol. 1, he took sex to be a "pre-given datum" upon which was "grafted" discursive and institutional formations of sexuality.[53] Foucault reworked his notion of body (and sex) such that it becomes a heterogeneous ensemble, utterly overlaid by the "apparatus of sexuality." Its overlay is not a layer to be peeled off, as was suggested by his described first draft. In other words, Foucault himself was tempted to formulate his work according to (2), but in the end he opted for version (3).

The difficulty, then, is to capture the relationship between these two factors. At the end of *The History of Sexuality,* vol. 1, Foucault moots an objection to his work: that he ignores the substance of the body (sex), in favor of something purely discursive (sexuality). Let me cite his response in some detail as an interesting attempt to deal with and characterize the problem:

> Here we need to distinguish between two questions. First, does the analysis of sexuality necessarily imply the *elision* of the body, anatomy, the biological, the functional? To this question, I think we can reply in the negative. In any case, the purpose of the present study is in fact to show how deployments of power are directly connected to the body—to bodies, functions, physiological processes, sensations, and pleasures; far from the body having to be effaced, *what is needed is to make it visible through an analysis in which the biological and the historical . . . are bound together in*

an increasingly complex fashion in accordance with the development of modern technologies that take life as their objective.[54]

Foucault refuses to accept the notion of sex *in itself.* His aim is to render the body visible through analyses that conjoin the historical and the biological. Whether Foucault succeeds or not in this, the formulation signifies a desire to achieve a version of (3), to come to terms with the inextricability of matter and its inscription.

Foucault's use of the term, visible, is interesting. Ironically, it bespeaks the very kind of analytic "gaze" that he is so often concerned to reveal. It suggests a kind of looking on, looking at the body, from the outside. Is this to privilege sight over and above other senses?[55] What motivates me here is a sense in which it is possible to listen to and learn from the body. I do not want to claim knowledge of the body outside but within discourse. There is much to be learned by paying attention to the body's character *as it is manifested through* the forms of inscription. If Foucault is right, inscription is something that occurs outside consciousness which becomes internalized, felt psychically and corporeally. This is OK as a starting point. However, I want to argue that a number of strategies are available to explore the limits and possibilities of inscription and its corporeal character via a mobile and changing sense of the body.[56]

First, I think that a sense of bodily revision and understanding can occur via what Elizabeth Grosz describes as "counterstrategic reinscription."[57] This represents a sense of change and bodily knowledge via a new and critical form of inscription. Perhaps Irigaray's writings on the two lips could be understood as a strategic attempt to reinscribe the female body, against the Freudian/Lacanian notion of female lack. Irigaray has written a paper, "When our lips speak together," in which she uses the image of the labia, two lips of the genitalia, which are constantly touching each other, one yet two, even multiple.[58] This metaphor of two lips can be contrasted either against Freud's notion of woman as lacking or against the single, male phallus—only one, never two, never many. Rather than an appeal to an essentialist biologism (women's bodies are found with the labia as a biological given), Irigaray's work can be seen as an inscriptive attempt to constitute a mapping of the female body which resists the Freudian/Lacanian production of woman as lack (counterstrategic). The multiplicity of Irigaray's femininity is a resistance to an undesirable singularity: lack, an identity defined by comparison to masculine morphology, and a freeing up of possibilities for the female body.

Second, I want to introduce another term, that of *practice*. The inscriptive account can be interpreted to render the body too passive. It isn't. And I don't think that Grosz's term, *counterstrategic reinscription,* is enough in that re-inscription suggests *another* process of inscription strategically developed to counter a form of dominance. Such moves are obviously crucial, e.g., in recon-stituting new forms of masculinity and femininity. But what about the body itself? Is it condemned to inscription and nothing else? Grosz recognizes and includes the physical body as that which is inscribed. It is both surface and substance which I think is a definite improvement. But it is still inert. If not dead meat, it's passive flesh. A flesh whose possibilities are always inscribed upon it, whether by the dominant culture or a resistant feminist politics. But inscription is only effected through constituting lived bodily experience, that is, through an interaction, an activity that occurs between substance, surface, and inscription. I introduce a notion of *practice* as a factor in bodily determination in order to signify an ongoing and variable process of embodiment and to represent that interaction.

The focus on practice is an attempt to highlight the milieu and process by which inscription could be said to occur. It is also an attempt to look at the activities of the body in this process. Let me suggest three metaphors as a means to exploring the body's role here.

1. One can imagine inscription as something that occurs on the dissecting table (prevalent in *Gray's Anatomy*): a dead body plus some grid projected onto it. A merit of this image is in the fact that some forms of inscription are given—for example, we find ourselves already with many forms of masculinity and femininity inscribed upon us. This is also the case in relation to many aspects of our sociality.

2. I have another image of the (dead) body sitting up and describing, or per-haps with others, constructing another grid, another mode of inscription. And then what? Lying down again to get another "dose" of inscription, this time determined by the (collective, counterstrategic) subject?

3. My next image is of a moving body, whose movements themselves (prac-tices) bespeak yet another grid which takes shape *as the body moves.* More fluid, perhaps holographic, these images depend on the body's practices to take form.[59] There is here a mutuality of form, a dialogue between substance and surface. I say they are in dialogue with each other because bodies cannot do anything. They are not phantasmagoria. This is represented by the fact

that the body *takes shape* in the context of the inscriptive process. It has form, albeit a fluid and changing one. Its taking shape is melded to the projection of the image itself. If the body were to have a pre-given substance, one could imagine a slide projector throwing an image upon an already formed body. The holographic nature of the projection here indicates the three-dimensionality of the projection itself; its corporeality as projection (and vice versa). The dialogue between substance and surface is an ongoing exchange, one that I conceive of in terms of practice.

One context I have in mind for (3) is the kind of dance/movement oriented to the creation of new movement possibilities, therefore involving an ongoing dialogue with a shifting and changing body. It is in such a context that the dancer and teacher Margaret Lasica speaks of working toward "an ever increasing vocabulary of the body."[60] Here the range of bodily movements, qualities, and senses of embodiment are posited as a shifting set of possibilities. These "possibilities" are brought to light, brought into bodily being, through the practices of movement itself. They are not pre-given as an inherent set of possibilities nor as an utterly open set of alternatives. Hence, the changing form of the body. The body responds to the accomplishment, the experience, of different forms of movement, which in turn embody different forms of potentiality. By this I mean that moving our bodies in particular kinds of ways enables and creates certain kinds of body. Working with a lot of muscular tension tends to produce rigid kinds of movement, for it helps develop an ability to perform such moves and does not train the body to work in other ways. There are some moves that a rigid body cannot perform, that require a certain amount of letting go. These require an ability to move in a lighter, more relaxed manner. In fact, all moving requires degrees of strength and hold in the body as well as degrees and regions of not holding. Working with too little strength or too much tension will not enable the performance of certain kinds of moves. Two extremes are utter rigidity and total release, although there are various qualities of hold, which suggests that the extremes do not occur at either end of one axis of movement analysis. The different qualities of movement and their associated bodily forms enable particular corporeal practices. The qualities of movement constitute a form or character of embodiment.

Ballet, for example, calls for an upright, centered, somewhat rigid approach. The drill of a ballet routine creates a habitual mode of "attacking" a move. That centered strength can empower a centered strong move. This would be useful if it can be called on rather than automatically assumed. Similarly, if unnecessary tension is released, and lengthening moves are practiced, then other sorts of moves become possible. The more discrimination of qualities of movement practiced, the more moves might "come to hand."[61] The point I am trying to make is that the sort of movement a body engages in will contribute to the future moves that it is able to carry out. Movement styles and bodily character do not come from nowhere. They have histories—both long term and short. I do not want to overstate the case, however: these histories are not already written upon each body. There is a sense in which they are emergent and emerging.

The above are rather functional terms of description, but imagery and imagination are also major factors of embodiment and its possibilities. This is now used in competitive sports, where visualization and imagination are seen to influence actualization. There are numerous other bodily qualities of movement that lend further possibility to the body. Bodily possibility also varies from moment to moment. The "same" body may feel very different over time, in different places, and according to different emotional states.

What possibilities of embodiment arise depend on the forms of practice themselves, the insights that guide them, and the knowledges that inform them.

Practice represents an active, shifting, though not unlimited, set of movements and forms of embodiment. A history of practice has an influence on the kinds of possibilities it can encompass. It also influences the shape and timber of embodiment. Practice is in turn affected by psychical and social configurations. Iris Marion Young has written a fascinating paper, "Throwing Like a Girl," on female bodily comportment which arises, as she sees it, from a "lack of practice in using the body in performing tasks."[62] She gives a number of idealized descriptions of the way women use their bodies, the bodily way in which female subjectivity is lived and practiced in Western, capitalist, urban society. For Young, sexual specificity engenders a certain kind of practice and therefore embodiment.

Practice is also able to limit movement, emotional, and bodily possibilities via habit, tension, holding patterns, and psyche. There is some written work on these matters.[63] For Kurtz and Prestera, the body comes to exhibit the psychic reality of the individual, and this can be seen in the ways the body is held, placed, and lived. Eventually, holding patterns become part of the person's habitual body character, the body's posture and im(mobility). There are also emotional investments in the body that shape its form.

For example, according to Kurtz and Prestera, in the overexpanded chest, "we find a fear of taking in energy from the outside, which involves the energy of relationships. The fear is one of softening, letting down one's guard, letting up one's pace."[64] Here the body's anatomy becomes a surface for a psychological form of inscription. Whether that psyche is in turn informed by social and cultural factors will depend on the way in which psychology is elaborated. I resist a psychology that ignores social and cultural determinants, but I also acknowledge that people negotiate individual responses to psychosocial complexities. Kurz and Prestera presume a universal, cross-cultural language of psychic manifestation in the body. The tendency to ignore cultural specificity or to falsely universalize clearly requires critical consideration. Young is careful to point out the cultural specificity of her observations.[65] Feldenkrais and Alexander do not develop a universal code of bodily language.

For all the mentioned bodyworkers, however, the possibilities for revision have to do with *shifting* these holding patterns and enabling a greater range of movement and other possibilities. Feldenkrais regards sensation, feeling, thought, and movement as connected terms of experience so a shift in one aspect will have resonances at other levels. This I see also as a form of reinscription, perhaps produced (if not derived) on an individual level. In order to reinscribe a body in this respect, the subject needs to learn to move differently, to move beyond his/her habitual modes: "Change involves carrying out an activity against the habit of life."[66] Bodyworkers operate in various ways to enable their subjects to interact with and shift their habitual limitations. Deep massage, for example, works on the fascia of muscle groups to release their habitual hold and shape to allow for different kinds of movement.

In sum, practice is an activity of the individual body/person. It may be culturally or collectively engendered, the result of bodywork or healing, form part of an artistic endeavor—or any combination of these. The creative, active body does not come from nowhere. In that sense, I think the body is both inscribed by a number of discourses, and is the possible subject of new practices which, in turn, create new forms of embodiment, and, if you like, reinscription. This is a sense of reinscription where the body/self participates in and is not merely subject of that reinscription. This is not necessarily to posit some underlying bodily essence that directs these forms of practice, for their results may exist beyond their conception. The subject of these practices is not merely a culturally determined somatic surface but also a present and changing bodily subjectivity.

Ethical implications

By now it should be fairly clear that I hold to no single account of the body; think that discourses inscribe bodies but do not totally produce them; and deem that bodies have a substance, a materiality, which can be explored through practice and altered in a number of ways, always within a discursive setting. I'd be interested to see a medical ethics develop which took account of the sense in which bodies are discursively produced, are culturally inscribed, and have a part to play in the determination of their own bodily and human being. Certainly there are generalized aspects of those forms of being, but the discursive milieu mitigates against any assertion of independent and immutable universality. To that extent, the medical epistemology may require modification. The modification of universality also pertains to ethics. Remember Ros Diprose's view, that ethics is a situated, embodied set of questions.[67] To explore and determine issues of medical ethics will require a sensitivity to the cultural and discursive setting of the subjects involved—as patients, theorists, doctors, and others. It may also be useful to inquire into the kinds of bodies assumed, involved, or posited.

Sometimes there will be a clash of cultures (e.g., Western medicine and Australian Aboriginal culture) where an ethics of imposition and a sensitivity to domination will need to extend to alternative and perhaps competing notions of the body and medical practices. Saggers and Gray write of the many failings of white, mainstream health services for Aborigines and the establishment of Aboriginal Health Services, staffed mainly by Aborigines. They refer to the difficulties that arise in relation to *two-way medicine,* that is, combining Western and traditional Aboriginal medicine. One of the problems has to do with the "differential power relation between practitioners of Western and Aboriginal medicine," their respective cultural settings, and the institutional bodies involved.[68] They write that any "solution" to these problems needs to be worked out by Aboriginal people themselves: "It may well be, as Nathan and Japanangka (1983) suggest, that allowing the two systems to exist side by side would serve the Aboriginal interest better."[69] This is not merely incommensurability, but a complexity of difference which arises from domination and colonization.

There is also the question of the passivity of the body, whether it is the result of medical "expertise," imposition, or the productions of inscription. Here I support the exploration of strategies that aim toward a greater participation of subjects in the re-creation of their own bodily and health possibilities. Bodies are not merely active agents, but neither are they passive recipients. Medical ethics is one means of negotiating that divide.

Notes

I would like to thank Ros Diprose for her careful comments and communication on an earlier draft of this paper, Paul Komesaroff for his encouragement and feedback, and those other contributors to this collection who also provided me with some very helpful comments. I am particularly indebted to Margaret Lasica for her ongoing generosity, curiosity, and teaching in relation to dance and the body. I owe many of my corporeal insights to her, although she bears no responsibility for their articulation here. Moving is one thing, writing about it is another. I would also like to thank Robert Young, deep-tissue therapist, for his "hands-on" advice and generous clarification on bodily matters.

1   W. Gibson, *Neuromancer* (London: Grafton Books, 1984), p. 76.

2   Ibid.

3   Ibid., p. 97.

4   Ibid., p. 67.

5   Ibid., p. 71.

6   R. Diprose, "A 'genethics' that makes sense," in R. Diprose and R. Ferrell, *Cartographies, Poststructuralism and the Mapping of Bodies and Spaces* (Sydney: Allen and Unwin, 1991). See also Diprose's contribution to this volume.

7   M. Gatens, *Feminism and Philosophy, Perspectives on Difference and Equality* (Oxford: Polity, 1991); E. Gross, "Philosophy, Subjectivity and the Body: Kristeva and Irigaray," in C. Pateman and E. Gross, eds., *Feminist Challenges, Social and Political Theory* (Sydney: Allen and Unwin, 1986); L. Irigaray, *This Sex which Is Not One,* trans. C. Porter and C. Burke (Ithaca, N.Y.: Cornell University Press, 1985); A. Jaggar and S. Bordo, *Gender/Body/Knowledge, Feminist Reconstructions of Being and Knowing* (New Brunswick and London: Rutgers University Press, 1989).

8   *Gray's Anatomy,* 15th ed. (London: Chancellor, 1858).

9   T. James, "The Ins and Outs of Natural Therapies," *Australian Doctor Weekly,* 24 April 1992, p. 27.

10   R. Rorty, *Philosophy and the Mirror of Nature* (Oxford, Basil Blackwell, 1980).

11   See for example M. Foucault, *The Birth of the Clinic, An Archeology of Medical Perception* (London: Vintage, 1975).

12   See for example E. Grosz, *Sexual Subversions: Three French Feminists* (Sydney: Allen and Unwin, 1989); Irigaray, *This Sex which Is Not One*; J. Kristeva, *Desire in Language: A Semiotic Approach to Literature and Art* (New York: Columbia University Press, 1980); T. Brennan, *Between Psychoanalysis and Feminism* (London and New York: Routledge, 1989); and Gatens, *Feminism and Philosophy.*

13   R. Braidotti, "Ethics Revisited: Women and/in Philosophy," in Pateman and Gross, *Feminist Challenges,* p. 48.

14   The same point can be made regarding the intransitivity of the experience of oppression. The suggestion is that to be oppressed "as a woman" will not simply translate into an understanding of what it is like to be oppressed "as a black" (C. Gallagher, "Marxism and the New

Historicism," in H. Aram Veeser, ed., *The New Historicism* [London and New York: Routledge, 1989]). The situation is even more complex in that someone may be oppressed as "a black woman," and this will not necessarily be an addition of the two separate experiences of oppression in terms of color and gender (M. T. Trinh, *Woman, Native, Other* [Bloomington: Indiana University Press, 1989]). For a more detailed discussion of this matter, see P. Rothfield, "Alternative Epistemologies, Politics and Feminism," *Social Analysis* 30 (1991), pp. 54–68.

15   M. Trinh, *Woman, Native, Other,* pp. 82–83.

16   A. Ong, "Colonialism and Modernity: Feminist Re-presentations of Women in non-Western Societies," *Inscriptions* 3/4, (1988), pp. 79–93, 84.

17   E. Said, *Orientalism* (London: Penguin, 1978).

18   D. Chakrabarty, "Postcoloniality and the Artifice of History: Who Speaks for "Indian" Pasts?", *Representations* 37 (Winter 1992).

19   For an interesting critique of the all-encompassing perspective, and an attempt to develop a "situated" sense of knowledge, see D. Haraway, "Situated Knowledges: The Science Question in Feminism and the Privilege of Partial Perspective," *Feminist Studies* 14, no. 3 (1988): 575–599.

20   M. Gatens, "A Critique of the Sex/Gender Distinction," in *Beyond Marxism* (Sydney: Intervention Publications). Reprinted in S. Gunew, ed., *A Reader in Feminist Knowledge* (London and New York: Routledge, 1983), pp. 148–150.

21   E. Grosz, "Notes towards a Corporeal Feminism," *Australian Feminist Studies* 5 (summer 1987): 1–16, 9.

22   Ibid., 10.

23   M. Feldenkrais, *Awareness through Movement* (Harmondsworth: Arkana Books, [1972] 1990), p. 60. Emphasis in original.

24   There are some who might describe this approach as realist.

25   A term whose etymology derives from Jean Baudrillard. See Chakrabarty, "Postcoloniality and the Artifice of History," p. 1.

26   It arises in part from Saussure's linguistic claim that meaning is a product of the language system. Saussure makes no use of any notion of reference (or truth for that matter) in his account of language, speech, and meaning. Thus, the world (ontology) does not take part in the construction of meaning—which is said to arise purely in terms of difference and participation within the language system. Through Marxist and feminist adaptations, questions of ontology have been reintroduced whereby Saussure's arbitrary constructions of language and representation create a reality that both serves particular political interests and is able to be challenged (S. Hall, "Recent Developments in Theories of Language and Ideology: A Critical Note," in S. Hall, D. Hobson et al., eds., *Culture, Media and Language* [London: Hutchinson, 1980]). Through the developments of poststructuralism, the systematicity of language or, more generally, signifying systems has been interrogated and relativized, so that linguistic systems have been taken to be more historical and local in their operations (D. Macdonell, *Theories of Discourse: An Introduction* [Oxford and New York: Blackwell, 1986]). Saussure and semiotics represent only one strand of thought associated with the productivist outlook. Other theorists would put the matter differently.

27   M. Foucault, *Power/Knowledge, Selected Interviews and Other Writings 1972–1977,* ed. C. Gordon (Brighton: Haverster, 1980), p. 112.

28   M. Foucault, *Discipline and Punish: The Birth of the Prison,* trans. A. Sheridan (Harmonds-worth: Penguin, [1975] 1977), pp. 19, 23.

29   Ibid. This point of Foucault's is also an argument against the notion of power as something that either limits freedom, comes from the outside, or is the power to do something. For Foucault, power is also productive: it produces something.

30   See L. Althusser (1970), "Ideology and Ideological State Apparatuses," in *Lenin and Philosophy,* trans. B. Brewster (New York: Monthly Review Press).

31   J. Henriques, W. Hollway et al., *Changing the Subject, Psychology, Social Regulation and Subjectivity* (London and New York: Methuen, 1984).

32   Gatens, "Critique of the Sex/Gender Distinction."

33   Foucault, *Power/Knowledge,* p. 58.

34   E. Grosz, "Inscriptions and Body-Maps: Representations and the Corporeal," in T. Threadgold and A. Cranny-Francis, eds., *Feminine Masculine and Representation* (Sydney: Allen and Unwin, 1990).

35   Gatens, "Critique of the Sex/Gender Distinction," p. 150.

36   Gatens first published this piece in 1983 and might not make her point in the same way today. I use this quotation as an illustration of a certain attitude toward the "physical," "anatomical" body.

37   V. Kirby, "Corpus delecti: The Body at the Scene of Writing," in R. Diprose and R. Ferrell, eds., *Cartographies, Poststructuralism and the Mapping of Bodies and Spaces* (Sydney: Allen and Unwin, 1991).

38   Ibid., p. 91.

39   Ibid., p. 146.

40   R. Braidotti, "The Politics of Ontological Difference," in T. Brennan, *Between Psychoanalysis and Feminism.*

41   Kirby, "Corpus delecti," p. 143.

42   E. Probyn, "The Body which Is Not One: Speaking an Embodied Self," *Hypatia* 6, no. 3 (fall 1991): 111–124, 112.

43   L. Wittgenstein, *Philosophical Investigations* (Oxford: Basil Blackwell, [1953] 1974).

44   Foucault, *Birth of the Clinic,* 146.

45   In the film *Flatliners,* medical students tried to understand more about human being/life by taking themselves near death, as if the *dead* body provides the secret to life. The setting of the "experiments" the students conduct is in a kind of mausoleum; their major subjects are anatomy and dissection.

46   A. Olsen, *Body Stories: A Guide to Experiential Anatomy* (New York: Station Hill Press, 1991), p. 39.

47   G. E. Moore, "A Defence of Common Sense," in *Philosophical Papers* (London: Allen and Unwin, 1959).

48   L. Wittgenstein, *On Certainty* (Oxford: Basil Blackwell, [1969] 1974), 10e and 12e.

49   Alexander's work shows that people embody perceptions, sensations, and forms of coordination which seem right to them but are very distorted. He writes of the little girl who had been unable to walk for some years upon learning to walk in a relatively straight manner, crying to her mother that she had been "*pulled out of shape*" (M. Alexander, *The Alexander Technique,*

selected and introduced by Edward Maisel [New York: Carol Communications, 1967], p. 17). He writes that it is crucial to engage with the subject's own perceptions and experience of bodily movement, that *argument* about the matter is inadequate: "He gets what he feels is the right position, but when he has an imperfect co-ordination he is only getting a position which fits with his defective co-ordination" (ibid., p. 11).

50   Anatomy could be explained according to either paradigm. In anatomy, the body is dissected, systematized, and theorized as a spatially mapped entity. According to Foucault, the anatomical body is the result of a certain kind of gaze that is traced through the eighteenth century, one which arose through the relaxation of religious taboos regarding opening up corpses. He writes of the gaze, the "grid" within which the known object (the body) appears, and the position the subject must occupy in order to map its elements (Foucault, *Birth of the Clinic*, p. 137). The story could be told in other ways—that is, that once the body could be opened up, its details were discovered, documented, and formulated into what has become modern anatomy. In the former story, the anatomical body is a made object; in the latter, a found object.

51   Grosz, "Inscriptions and Body-Maps," 62.

52   Ibid., p. 71.

53   Foucault, *Power/Knowledge*, p. 210.

54   M. Foucault, *History of Sexuality*, vol. 1: An Introduction, trans. R. Hurley (Harmondsworth: Penguin, 1978), pp. 151–152. My emphases.

55   It seems to me that an aspect of the problems associated with body image derive from a visually dominated notion of the female body—that it must *look* thin (from the outside). This norm then becomes internalized so that women develop a highly distorted vision of themselves, of a body image that derives from a look from the outside. A dominance of vision also manifests in aerobics where the contours of a lycra-clad body function as a measure of "success." This is so divorced from a sense of bodily well-being that it is quite acceptable to feel pain in order to achieve (visual) "gain." Vicki Kirby writes of the body as a corporeal envelope (Kirby, "Corpus delecti," p. 88). Isn't it more a package?

56   Notice the ambiguity between sense as definition or concept and sense as feeling. In relation to the body, it may be prudent to include both elements.

57   Grosz, "Inscriptions and Body-Maps," p. 64.

58   Irigaray, *This Sex which Is Not One*.

59   I am indebted to Robert Young for the suggestion that the body is holographic.

60   Personal communication 1991.

61   I use this locution advisedly, to recall its different context of articulation—where coming to hand was seen to imply a realistic form of reference (Probyn, "Body which Is Not One"). Notice that here it is an evolving, undetermined (not indeterminate) unfolding. Probyn, in the same article, refers to Deleuze's work on the body as a pleat (or number of pleats) whose folding and unfolding sustains and inverts the inside/outside distinctions of the body.

62   I. M. Young, "Throwing Like a Girl: A Phenomenology of Feminine Body Comportment, Motility and Spatiality," in I. M. Young and J. Allen, eds. *The Thinking Muse: Feminism and Modern French Philosophy* (Bloomington: Indiana University Press, 1989), p. 58.

63   Alexander, *Alexander Technique*; Feldenkrais, *Awareness through Movement*; R. Kurtz and

H. Prestera, *The Body Reveal: What Your Body Says about You* (San Francisco: Harper and Row, 1976); and S. Keleman, *Emotional Anatomy* (Berkeley: Center Press, 1985).

64   Kurtz and Prestera, *Body Reveals*, p. 81.

65   Young, "Throwing Like a Girl," p. 53.

66   Alexander, *Alexander Technique*, p. 3.

67   Diprose, " 'Genethics' that Makes Sense."

68   S. Saggers and D. Gray, *Aboriginal Health and Society: The Traditional and Contemporary Aboriginal Struggle for Better Health* (Sydney: Allen and Unwin, 1991), p. 150.

69   Ibid., p. 151.

The body biomedical ethics forgets

Rosalyn Diprose

There is a curious silence which resounds throughout discussions of the ethics of biomedicine. One rarely finds mention of the body, despite what would seem to be obvious: the object of biomedical theory and practice is the body. What prescriptive and normative ethics assumes it regulates is not so much the relation between biomedicine and bodies but the relation between biomedicine and autonomous, disembodied individuals. I will argue here that biomedical ethics, in forgetting the body, misconceives both the nature of the individual and the nature of the relation between the individual and biomedicine. In its forgetfulness, and armed with its universal rules, biomedical ethics runs the risk of being at best ineffective and at worst unethical. This risk is perhaps no better illustrated in the first instance than by debates about the ethics of reproductive practices such as surrogacy.

Principles of biomedical ethics

In 1990 the Australian National Bioethics Consultative Committee (NBCC), published a report on surrogacy. This report stands out as a measured analysis of the area, attempting as it does to steer a course between those who oppose surrogacy in any form and those who view it as a legitimate expression of a woman's right to participate in projects of her choice.[1] It also provides a useful guide to what is typically taken to be the nature of the individual and of relations between individuals in applied biomedical ethics. Accordingly, this chapter will take the *Surrogacy Report* as its point of departure for a discussion of some of the major ethical issues associated with the area of surrogacy. (It should be noted that there are several difficulties with the term *surrogacy* that are discussed in the NBCC's report. For my purposes here, I take surrogacy to mean an arrangement in which a woman agrees to gestate a child for, and subsequently to relinquish it to, another person or persons.) The principles are spelled out in the report as follows:

1. *The principle of personal autonomy* or self-determination—namely, that people should have the right to make their own life decisions for themselves as long as those decisions do not involve harm to others;

2. *The principle of justice*—namely, that arrangements between individuals should not involve exploitation and should best serve the interests of all those involved (in this case those of the surrogate mother, the unborn child, and the commissioning couple);

3. *The principle of the common good*—namely, that the good of the whole community must be considered in arrangements made between individuals. (p. 14)

The NBCC is explicit about the kind of individual it assumes in its principle of autonomy. Following John Stuart Mill's essay *On Liberty,* the individual is defined by the basic tenet: "over himself, over his own body and mind the individual is sovereign" (p. 15). In the only direct reference to the body in its report, the NBCC attributes to it the status of a passive object governed by an individual agent who somehow stands above it. From then on this relation is assumed. *Autonomy* implies the freedom to decide how to dispose of one's body so long as others are not harmed by that decision. This is the concept of "negative freedom" as defined by Isaiah Berlin: the freedom from external constraint.[2] Both the biomedical practitioner and the bioethicist present a potential threat to the individual's negative freedom: the biomedical practitioner by gaining access to the agent's body, which may undermine her sovereignty over her body, and the ethicist by placing legal restrictions on what the individual can do with her body.

The authors of the report assume that the principles of justice and of the common good govern relations between individuals and refer back to the principle of autonomy and its assumptions about the body. They believe that the autonomous individual comes before her social relations with others and that hence her autonomy is separate from the spheres of justice and the common good. According to the NBCC, the ethicist must reconcile the principle of personal autonomy with those of justice and the common good. In this, the implicit focus of regulation is the relations of contract and exchange between isolated self-governing individuals, where the object of exchange is the individual's body.

This model of exchange is a natural one in a society structured around the idea of a market economy, where the body very easily assumes the status of property. The right of the individual to exchange his or her labor for financial reward is taken for granted. This amounts to the right to dispose of one's body, and the product of one's body, as one sees fit.[3] At the same time, ethical limits are placed upon ways in which the body can become a legitimate object of exchange. The value and integrity of the individual's body, as assumed by the individual himself or herself, is weighted against the value and integrity of others and of the body of the community. In the case of bioethics, the situation is complicated by the fact that biomedical science not only competes with the law for the right to dictate what should be done with the individual's body, at the expense of the individual's autonomy, but it also increases the options open to the individual in the exercise of his or her negative freedom.

I should like to develop this model of exchange further, now that I have made the position of the body explicit. In the case of surrogacy and in vitro fertilization (IVF), the object of exchange and regulation is a woman's body. Those players competing for sovereignty over this body are the woman herself (considered separate from her body), the unborn child, the family, the bioethicist (as representative of the law and the common good), and, in the case of IVF more so than surrogacy, the biomedical practitioner. The woman's autonomy (her right to sovereignty over her own body) is pitted against the possibility that her actions (and those of biomedical science) may bring harm to herself, to the child in the future, to others, and to the fabric of society in general.

It would seem, therefore, that reproductive practices are an issue for the bioethicist because the interests of other bodies, besides the maternal body, have to be considered. In fact, the NBCC goes so far as to imply that it is not just sovereignty over the woman's body that is of concern but also that of the child because, in the case of surrogacy, the child, rather than the mother's body, is the exchangeable commodity (p. 20). Such a suggestion, in keeping with the model of exchange, takes the pregnant body to be two bodies. Pregnancy as an ethical issue becomes a problem about competing claims between two individuals, the mother and the fetus, where both are assumed to be autonomous, self-governing entities with the right to sovereignty over their respective bodies (the mother in reality, the fetus potentially). There are two immediate problems with this assumption: the problem of the legitimacy of dividing the pregnant body in this way and, even if this legitimacy is granted, the problem of the decisions about whose rights should take priority, which become reduced to a question of whose side you are on. Personal preference necessarily creeps into an ethical decision-making process which purports to be an objective application of universal principles.

Besides the problematic assumption that we can divide the pregnant body into two autonomous entities, also questionable is the more general assumption of a distinction between the autonomous agent on the one hand and her body and the sphere of social relations on the other. For example, while the NBCC finds no problem with this distinction (p. 15), doubts about the notion of autonomy begin to undermine the model of exchange and regulation which this distinction supports. One submission to the NBCC which opposes surrogacy claims that for a decision to be autonomous, the agent must be fully informed of the consequences of that decision for her future well-being. Yet, in the case of surrogacy or IVF, a woman's future well-being is necessarily jeopardized (by the trauma of giving up her child, in the case of surrogacy, and by the trauma of the process and its possible failure, in the case of IVF). Hence, a woman's decision to be the object of such practices can never be fully informed or, therefore, autonomous.[4] This objection implies, among other things, that the distinction between the agent and her embodied well-being is illegitimate. Another submission claims that the patriarchal imperative to procreate and women's disadvantaged social position influences and limits the choices they can make, leaving them open to exploitation by the commissioning couple, in the case of surrogacy, and by biomedical science, in the case of IVF (p. 17).

To suggest that one's choices are determined to some extent by the values of the social context and one's social position questions the distinction between the sphere of personal autonomy on the one hand and a "common good" on the other. While the NBCC insists on the validity of such a distinction, it goes on, some pages later, to point out the necessary vagueness that surrounds the idea of "core values" which make up the "common good" in a liberal democratic society (p. 18). It suggests that the notion of personal autonomy is not so much in opposition to the common good but is one value that represents and defines our common good. In extending this suggestion we could conclude not only that the values that make up the "common good" have some bearing on the assumption of autonomy but also on the choices open to us in the exercise of our so-called freedom.

While going some way to challenge the notion of autonomy, these arguments conclude that women should be prevented from participating in such reproductive practices, in the interests of their own protection. Further restriction of women's action by the law is justified on the grounds that it prevents them from making ill-founded choices—choices that will further restrict their freedom and enhance their exploitation. This conclusion reinvokes the notion of autonomy. It inconsistently assumes that the ethicist, unlike the woman in question, knows ahead of time what her experience will be and it assumes that a woman is free (from patriarchal influences) if she keeps her body to herself. Other challenges to a notion of autonomous agency can be found elsewhere in the literature on biomedical ethics. Daniel Callahan, for example, argues that, while the assumption of autonomy is necessary in medical practice to uphold patient's rights, it does tend to diminish the sense of obligation others may have toward us, and vice versa.[5] Taken to its logical conclusion, the notion of the autonomous self discourages the ideal of community and interdependence and encourages a sterile and uncaring relationship between biomedical science and the individual.

Insofar as the principles of autonomy, justice, and the common good distance the agent from her body and from others, they are inadequate for dealing with the ethics of biomedical practice and result in pragmatic and fragile judgments. For example, the concern of the NBCC to protect the autonomy of the "surrogate" and the child leads it to conclude that surrogacy arrangements should be permitted under strict controls. In particular, advertising and surrogacy agencies should be controlled and, in view of the fact that a surrogacy contract could force a mother to give up her child, it decided such contrasts should not be enforceable. This conclusion is consistent with the view, which I have argued elsewhere, that while the surrogacy contract is unethical, surrogacy is not.[6] However, it is based on a model of autonomy as sovereignty over one's body and a contractual model of social relations, as a result of which it encounters two immediate problems. First, it upholds the ideal of social contracts between autonomous individuals while excluding pregnant women, thus reinforcing a tradition of sexual inequality that excludes women from public relations on the basis of their sex. Second, while emphasizing women's rights to do with their bodies what they will it has to face objections based on exactly the same ethical principles from opponents of surrogacy in any form who argue that even in informal surrogacy the surrogate's autonomy is not preserved, or the autonomy of the future child is threatened, or the values of the "common good" are at risk.

While ethical judgments based on these principles are I think ultimately incoherent, a certain pattern does emerge in them. I want to suggest that whether or not an activity is considered ethical depends not so much on questions of autonomy but rather on the significance of the body in question. Behind a veil of universal principles, what seems to be actually monitored by bioethics, implicitly rather than explicitly, is the extent to which the body can be altered, by whom, and to what end. What biomedical ethics seeks to preserve is the integrity of the body such that it remains compatible with the social body. It is ethical, therefore, to restore a diseased body to its former status as a publicly viable body, but it is unethical to change a body, say through genetic engineering, to the point where it cannot be accommodated or recognized by the social body. Pregnancy also involves a change in the integrity of the body. And perhaps it is because the pregnant body is considered a deviation from the norm, as well as the site of the reproduction of the "normal" body, that pregnancy becomes an ethical issue whether or not the body in question is caught up in explicitly controversial practices (such as surrogacy, abortion, IVF) or not. Even in "normal" pregnancy, what the mother does with her body—what she ingests, how she moves and when—is considered to be a legitimate target for moral concern. It would seem then that the labor of pregnancy does not enjoy the same freedom of exchange as the labor of the body in the marketplace (a point to which I will return later in this article). If it is necessary to abandon the principles of autonomy and justice in order to deal with the maternal body, then perhaps it is the principles rather than different bodies that require further scrutiny.

I do not seek to provide a more definitive view about the ethics of practices such as surrogacy than that of the NBCC, but I do hope to make explicit what is at stake in ethical discourse by locating the place of the body within it and by taking issue with the principles upon which current decisions are being made. It seems to me that the philosophical principles that form the basis of biomedical ethics are yet to catch up with the problems they are meant to address or the decision-making process they inform. There are at least two aspects of the model of exchange used in biomedical ethics which require closer scrutiny: the relationship between the individual and his or her body, and the relationship between the body on the one hand and biomedical science on the other.

The individual with a body

There is much to suggest that the body is not a simple passive object over which the individual has real or even potential control. In saying this I am not suggesting a return to a precritical notion of an innate biological complex which dictates our every move. Rather, I am suggesting that, as we are never without a body, a notion of an individual where the body is given the secondary status of an appendage subjected to property rights would seem to assume much while explaining little. It might just be possible that this body contributes to what we are in ways other than as a thing to be controlled.

In attempting to reinsert the body back into bioethics I'll begin with some apparent anomalies. In his entertaining book *The Man Who Mistook His Wife for a Hat,* neurologist Oliver Sacks describes cases where people think they have a limb where there is none and, conversely, where they think the limb they have belongs to someone else. There is the man who discovered someone else's leg in his bed but found, when he attempted to throw it out, that he somehow came after it.[7] When asked where his own leg might be, he replied, somewhat disconcertedly, that he had no idea—it seemed to have disappeared and been replaced by someone else's. Conversely, and more commonly, there is the phenomenon of the phantom limb where amputees experience their bodies as including a limb which is in fact missing.[8] The memory of the limb or the "limb-image" is so real to the amputee that he or she often experiences pain in that which is missing and, in all cases cannot use an artificial limb unless the phantom is real.

Now we could dismiss these examples of relations between an individual and his or her body as anomalies resulting from a psychological disorder which distorts the reality of the body. But as Sacks points out, these patients are, in all other respects, reasonable and clear headed. What these examples might suggest is that the individual has a particular relation to his or her body that is not accessible to the casual observer. Second, they suggest that illness or any radical change in the body represents a shift not only in one's experience of one's body (as if the body was separate from the self) but also in one's experience of one's self per se. Or, in the case of a phantom limb, there would seem to be a resistance to a change in the image of one's embodied self. It is not so much that the individual stands above his or her body in appreciation of its capacities and social significance but that the capacities of the body designate the individual's place in the world and, hence, his or her social identity.

These suggestions about the relation between the individual and the body can be applied to more commonplace changes in the texture of the body. Drew Leder describes the fracture in the structure of the self that can occur with the experience of pain. A man is playing tennis. He does not reflect on his body. His posture and movements are engaged with the environment without explicit thought or will. But a sudden sharp pain disrupts this immersed activity. He gives up the game, focusing instead on the well-being of his body. When his body becomes the focus of his attention, he can no longer use it. What turns out to be a heart attack is followed some time later by another, leading to profound changes in this man's social identity. Besides a reduction in capabilities, he experiences a shift in his relation to his body and to others. He is more self-conscious of his body, he anticipates pain, and the "everyday concerns of others recede as he finds himself thinking more frequently of death."[9]

What Leder provides, following Merleau-Ponty, is an account of the individual as *a lived body*. The body, in this model, is not in the first instance a discrete, unified entity which, under the direction of individual agency, is used as an instrument to engage with objects in the world outside it. Rather, in our ordinary, everyday activities, our body is open upon a world and engaged with it in such a way that we are hardly aware of this body at all. I do not direct my body to act. For the most part my body, and the world with which it is engaged, are not objects of my attention. This lived body is a complex field of activity which functions as an orientation center in relation to an environment. And while a reference point for my spatial orientation, this body is not something *I have*; it is what *I am* in my relation to objects and others. This body is at the same time absent from explicit awareness and present in order for me to be engaged with the world at all. This is the "ecstatic" body—the self dispersed and open to the world prior to the distinctions between mind and body, self and world, self and other: what some phenomenologists call the transcendent self, what Heidegger calls ecstatic dwelling in the world in the mode of comportment toward the ready to hand,[10] and what I have elsewhere described as the habitual body, the capacities of which have been constituted through a repetition of acts such that the self is at home with his or her body in the world in which it is dispersed.[11]

So Leder's tennis player is ecstatically engaged with the world. His body is absent, in the sense of being engaged in the world without his explicit awareness or control. Or, as Leder puts it: "The game is made possible only by this bodily self-concealment."[12] Yet his body is also present—the tennis player is his body, his body is the fabric of his being-in-the-world. With the onset on pain there is a tear in this fabric. This "affective call," as Leder terms it,[13] fundamentally alters the player's mode of being-in-the-world. The structure of the self is disrupted when part of the body becomes an object of attention such that normal functioning becomes impossible. It is not just the pain in itself which spoils the game: pain introduces a split between the mind and the body, the self and the world, the self and the other. Rather than dwelling with a body in a world with others, one's body, the world, and the other are placed at a distance. A breakdown in the operation of the body amounts to a collapse in the structure of the self. As this collapse involves internal limitations upon the self's capacity to act, it can be said to constrain the individual's "positive" freedom.[14]

There are at least three ways in which Leder's account of the embodied self challenges the liberal model of the individual used by the NBCC and in other instances of applied bioethics. First, the body is not so much an appendage to the self but is itself the locus of subjectivity—the very fabric of the self. Second, as the body is the locus of one's being-in-the-world, one's social identity is derived from one's particular activities and will vary in each case. The lived body expresses difference in identity. Finally, the distinction between the individual agent and the body over which she or he is sovereign—the distinction upon which the principle of autonomy is based—is a secondary and derivative mode of being in the world. For Leder, self-conscious intentionality, sovereignty over one's body, is a mode of existence that arises after a call back to one's body from habitual, ecstatic engagement in the world. Moreover, in this state of "having" rather than "being" a body, one is alienated from the world, from others, and from the self. In pain, and, it would seem, in biomedical ethics, one is alone with a body who is a stranger. Yet, if we throw the stranger out of bed we are sure to follow after it.

David Schenck follows the same phenomenological tradition as Leder, but takes Merleau-Ponty's account of the embodied self as a foundation for medical ethics. The body for Schenck is not just a center of activity by which we are engaged with our environment, but as such, the body is *literally our selves expressed.*[15] The body we are with is a kind of sign out there in the world inviting interpretation by, and response from, others. And it is this text of our being-in-the-world which is the object of biomedical practice. As medicine deals with what Schenck calls the "brokenness of bodies," it is dealing with the collapse of one's social expressiveness.[16] It is the fact that the body is the self expressed which gives medical practice its ethical dimension. A broken body invites care by others, and in this call for care one gives over to medical practitioners the responsibility for restoring the structure of the self.

These alternative accounts of the relation between the individual and his or her body suggest that any practice that perpetuates the alienation apparent in the distinctions between self and body, self and world, is unethical. Hence, the assumption in biomedical ethics that the body is merely an appendage to the self over which we ideally have sovereignty gives biomedical practice an unethical foundation. In the case of the so called "broken body," medicine assumes that this body is merely a thing which requires fixing, a malfunctioning object of secondary concern to the self. By attending to the body as if it were a thing rather than attending to its rehabituation, medicine risks doubling the objectification and alienation of the body inherent in its collapse. In this, the body, and therefore the self, remains a stranger. Biomedical ethics perpetuates this distinction between self and body in viewing its task as weighing up competing claims for sovereignty over a body. Insofar as it thus contributes to a fragmentation of one's being-in-the-world, biomedical ethics is unethical.

On the model of the self as a lived body, what is at stake in medical intervention is not so much the autonomy of the individual understood as negative freedom, sovereignty over one's body. What is at stake is the restoration of one's embodied being-in-the-world, one's positive freedom. And, what is at stake in medical practice is not the integrity of a passive object that is fundamentally universal in its nature. As the body is the texture of the self's social identity which varies in each case, what is at stake in medical practice is the identity of one's difference. The phenomenological model not only reinstates the dignity of the patient by stressing that the fabric upon which biomedicine works is the self, but it also highlights the specificity of that person's condition, however common that condition may appear to be. And, in claiming a difference in the identity of one's lived body, the model challenges the assumption of a common good (a set of interests applicable to any body) without abandoning that of concern to Callahan: the notion of community and its attendant obligation of care.

Biomedical science and the unbroken body

These accounts of the lived body go some way to challenge the foundations of biomedical ethics; however, there are several problems arising from the distinction between the ecstatic habitual body (the body's self-concealment in unimpeded activity) and the broken body (the disruption to the texture of subjectivity that occurs when the body's integrity is altered).

In the first place, not all changes to the texture of the body can or should be understood in terms of an inhibition of (positive) freedom, or, therefore, in terms of self-estrangement. Pregnancy, for example, obviously involves profound changes in bodily capacities, shape, and texture and a shift in the awareness of one's body. Yet, as Iris Young points out in her discussion of pregnant embodiment, pregnancy can hardly be described as a collapse of the structure of the self.[17] Insofar as phenomenologists formulate the experience of being thrown back onto an awareness of one's body exclusively in terms of disruption and alienation they miss much about how we ordinarily accommodate changes to our bodies.

While pregnancy may involve some disruption to the habitual body and some sense of invasion by a foreign body, this sense of alienation is as much a product of the social significance of pregnancy as the nonpregnant habitual body is a product of its engagement with the world. Young argues that pregnancy can be more constructively characterized as a mode of being that undermines the border between the inside and the outside of the body. In pregnancy it is not clear where one body ends and the other begins, nor is it clear where the pregnant body ends and the world begins. She suggests that pregnancy consists in an expansion of the borders of self rather than a collapse in the structure of the self. This change in the integrity of the body does not necessarily alienate one from the world. It does not precipitate a radical split between self and world in that the pregnant woman may find it difficult to negotiate the shifts in the border between herself and the world, but she negotiates it all the same. Nor does pregnancy simply alienate one from one's body: the pregnant body is "other" in the sense that it could be said to include another, but this other is also part of the self. In sum, Young characterizes pregnancy as an awareness of one's body which does not prohibit engaged activity. Pregnancy is a change in the integrity of the body which highlights the possibility of altering the structure of the self through rehabituation without the need to think of this in negative terms: in terms of a paralyzing division between self and world, self and other, self and body.

Insofar as bioethics conceives of the pregnant body as two discrete bodies in one, or any body as atomized and self contained, it overlooks the fundamental interdependence of self and world, self and other—an interdependence that is effected through the body. And insofar as both mainstream bioethics and phenomenology view a change in the body's integrity negatively, as disruption and a deviation from the norm, they cannot accommodate a possible flexibility in our being-in-the-world: the possibility of self-creativity in integrating corporeal changes. On the other hand, if we think of pregnancy as an example of a change in the integrity of one's body which accommodates another within an expansion of the self then we can explain what neither the mainstream bioethicist nor the phenomenologist can easily come to terms with: that a surrogate mother may begin by treating her body as an object of exchange but end by wanting to keep the product of her labor. To hold a surrogate to her contract, as some suggest, is to assume that the product of her labor is not part of herself. The same assumption, that corporeal changes cannot be accommodated by changes in the structure of the self, would have us cure amputees of their phantom limbs even though they cannot function without them. And I shudder to think what this assumption would have us do with a strange leg in our bed.

Another problem with the distinction between the body's self-concealment in free activity and disruption to the structure of self precipitated by changes in one's body is that it begs the question as to what determines the capacities and interests as well as the "social expressiveness" of the lived body before it is broken or before it expands. As I mentioned earlier, the literature on biomedical ethics contains some uncertainty about the notion of an autonomous self distinct from the values that make up the "common good," as if individual decisions are uncontaminated by those values. The phenomenological account of the lived body addresses this problem insofar as it claims that the lived body is constituted by its dwelling in the world. That is, the capacities and habits, and therefore the interests, of any body do not arise separately from the discourses and practices that make up the world in which it is engaged. The lived body is constituted through its engagement, through the everyday processes of habituation.[18] However, in their distinction between the habitual, ecstatic body, and the broken alienated body, some phenomenologists leave us with a problem as to where to place the work of biomedical science.

Schenck's analysis suggests that biomedical science only plays a part in the constitution of our embodied being-in-the-world after the body has broken. The ethics of biomedicine is thus restricted to its practice of altering bodies in the repair of our social expressiveness. But this incorrectly implies that biomedical science is not one of the discourses and practices that make up the world in which we dwell. Biomedicine is not just a practice that works directly on bodies. It is also a field of knowledge—and, as Michel Foucault suggests, there is no field of "knowledge that does not presuppose and constitute at the same time power relations."[19] Not only is biomedical science enmeshed within the values that constitute the so-called common good, but also it holds a privileged place in disseminating knowledge about what a body is, how it functions, and what its capabilities are. In this it delineates the normal body from the abnormal. So it is possible that biomedical science not only restores the body after a breakdown in the structure of the self but, as a field of knowledge, it may play a part in the constitution of that body prior to its alienation. Consequently, the ethics of biomedicine may be located not just within its practice of restoring our embodied being-in-the-world but also in that which determines our well-being.

This is a view based on Foucault's analyses of the relationship between power, knowledge, and the body. His view of the nature of this relationship is different from that of bioethics, based on universal principles, and phenomenology. As I have suggested, one of the principles upon which biomedical ethics is based is that of individual autonomy, where the concern is to minimize the power of both the law and biomedical science to limit the sovereignty we have over our bodies by placing external restrictions on our freedom. Schenck's and Leder's accounts of our embodied being-in-the-world favors an almost opposite conclusion: the ethics of biomedicine rests on its power to restore the self, the "positive" freedom of which has been restricted through a breakdown in the body. The power of biomedicine in this account is a precondition to freedom, providing the medical practitioner takes care not to intensify the alienation inherent in the collapse in the structure of the self.

Foucault lines up with a phenomenological account of freedom insofar as he suggests that only in extreme cases is power exercised to constrain or forbid actions. He defines power as a mode of government, where to govern means "to structure the possible field of action of others."[20] And he says that, if power governs possible actions then it must be exercised over free subjects—that is, subjects who are faced with a range of possible actions and have the ability to choose between them. So power is not opposed to freedom: power operates to determine what actions are open to the individual. In this sense Foucault would agree with the conclusion of Schenck's and Leder's analyses that restoring a body's capacities amounts to restoring its freedom to act. But Foucault's analysis goes further. As he is concerned with how power operates to structure a possible field of actions, he pays attention to how individuals gain the ability to act in certain ways prior to any perceived breakdown. As Paul Patton suggests in his analysis of Foucault's account of power and freedom, both the concept of positive freedom (the absence of internal constraints) and that of negative freedom (the absence of external constraints) presuppose the capacity to act.[21] Foucault is concerned with how these capacities are determined by the operation of power.

Foucault claims that power is not so much prohibitive but productive at a material level, that is, at the level of the body. In his later work he attempts to answer the following question: "What mode of investment of the body is necessary and adequate for the functioning of a capitalist society such as ours? . . . One needs to study what kind of body the current society needs."[22] His claim is that bodies are made, not given, and that they are made to fit within a certain social structure. Bodies are a product of historically specific knowledges and social practices which invest the body with power—with the power to act in certain ways.

What Foucault finds in his own study of what kind of body our society needs is the operation of what he calls microtechniques of power which constitute individuals within a political and economic field of domination and control.

This almost invisible operation of power, which he sometimes calls "pastoral power," is based on a political rationality that promotes the health and welfare of the individual to ensure the welfare of the whole.[23] This is the mode of government of the individual which is endorsed by an ethics that seeks to uphold the "common good": attending to our health and welfare does not require laws that restrict actions, it is not seen as a restriction of freedom or therefore an exercise of power. But, according to Foucault, this ethicopolitical rationality embraces an operation of power that delimits our freedom to act. It distributes techniques of power through knowledges and certain social practices which operate on the body to transform it, divide it, invest it with capacities, and train it to perform certain functions.[24] This is the operation of power which constitutes our embodied being in the world.

Health and power

Contrary to Schenck's account, Foucault finds that modern science and medicine play a vital role in this everyday constitution of bodies prior to their breakdown. He claims that "the health and physical well-being of the population" emerged in the eighteenth and nineteenth centuries "as one of the essential objectives of political power."[25] The nexus between health and political power arose through concern over the maintenance of a productive labor force. As a consequence, biomedical science has emerged entangled with other knowledges and practices which effectively divide bodies around a norm. The healthy are divided from the unhealthy in terms of what is useful and what is "less amenable to profitable investment."[26] The health of bodies has become a question of economic management: we are subjected through our bodies via an operation of power aimed, more or less, at the production of individuals who are useful to our economic structure. The individual subject is produced through this operation of power in two senses: he or she is subjected to the actions of others and attains a social identity, or, in Schenck's terms, a social expressiveness.[27]

According to Foucault's analysis there are at least three techniques of power that operate through knowledges and practices such as biomedical science: discipline, surveillance, and confession. Discipline proceeds through supervision, the collection of data about individual performance, and a system of penalties and corrections. The everyday supervision of pregnancy, and the dissemination of information about it, would be one current example of the way discipline combines with surveillance and the production of knowledge in biomedicine. This operation of power is normalizing in that discipline and surveillance assume normal categories and through these practices we measure ourselves against these norms and regulate ourselves accordingly. And surveillance, categorization and normalization have material effects. Individual bodies are objects of this operation of power—they attain a limited range of capacities, and they become docile and productive under its exercise. And they are the instruments of power in that they become complicit in the discipline and surveillance of both themselves and others.[28] There is no need for laws to restrict our activity: our activity is already restricted through a mode of government that trains bodies capable of a socially prescribed range of activities.

While the political investment of different bodies and different parts of a body is normalizing, it is not uniform.[29] Our social practices not only produce docile, self-regulating bodies but integrate these into a hierarchy of domination, control, and mutual dependence. The pregnant woman is subjected to more public scrutiny than the medical practitioner who directly monitors her. The power relation is asymmetrical. Yet, neither party can easily extract itself from this relation without attracting the condemnation of the community.

This normalization of bodies also relies on the technology of confession. We are in the habit of confessing what we assume to be the truth of our health, desires, crimes, and sexuality which serves to mark us out further for surveillance and correction. This aspect of Foucault's analysis suggests that, while biomedicine exercises power by structuring the possible field of our actions, we will have difficulty locating there a single, intentional agent of power. Biomedicine reproduces, rather than invents or enforces singlehandedly, the norms and assumptions that pervade all our social practices. Nor are we forced to subject ourselves to medical attention. We are complicit in our subjection in that, for the most part, we willingly submit ourselves to the techniques of discipline and surveillance that determine the possibilities open to us in the exercise of our freedom, in the body's self-concealment in free activity.

The relationship between biomedical science and the body would seem to be far more complex than either biomedical ethics or phenomenology assumes. Foucault's analysis of the relation between power, knowledge, and the body suggests a continuum, with regard to constitutive effects, between biomedical practice (and its ability to alter the body in order to restore the self) and biomedicine as a field of knowledge (and its place within a disciplinary network which makes us what we are). Without the need for coercion or prohibitions, biomedicine, both as a practice and a field of knowledge, joins forces with other disciplines to reproduce an economically productive and efficient social body which marginalizes certain bodies and which maintains asymmetrical power relations. For the most part, biomedical ethics, intent on locating external restrictions to freedom and autonomy, misses much of the work of biomedical science in the reproduction of asymmetrical power relations.

The process of the habituation and normalization of bodies begins at birth, if not before, which would explain why the pregnant body, in all its forms, as the site of the reproduction of the social body, attracts more than its fair share of moral attention. As Foucault has attempted to show, in the medical politics which arose in the eighteenth century, the family became "the first and most important instance for the medicalisation of individuals. The family is assigned a linking role between general objectives regarding the good health of the social body and individuals' desire or need for care."[30] Without denying that the moral concern about pregnancy is motivated by a genuine consideration for the health and well-being of mothers and their children, it is also consistent with the political investment of "healthy," productive bodies suitable for exchange in a labor market.

At the same time, the pregnant body, while apparently the target for unlimited surveillance, is itself anomalous in the labor market it reproduces. As Moira Gatens argues, from the time of its inception the social contract has implicitly or explicitly excluded the labor of women's bodies from the realm of sociopolitical freedom.[31] Woman's labor has been privatized and the product of her labor has traditionally been viewed as belonging to someone else. The labor of pregnancy has also been privatized but remains, paradoxically, open to public scrutiny in the interests of the health and welfare of the social body. Of course, feminism has attempted, with some success, to extend the principles of "free contract and exchange" to women and, in this context, the apparent proliferation and commercialization of surrogacy, should not be a surprising by-product. But, while women's labor is no longer explicitly excluded from the body politic, pregnancy remains foreign to the social contract for the reasons given. It would seem, then, that recent concerns about the ethics of surrogacy and IVF emerge as an extension of an all-pervasive regime of surveillance concerned with the reproduction of the social body. Again, without denying that opposition to practices like surrogacy and IVF have women's well-being at heart, such opposition inadvertently joins forces with other disciplinary regimes involved in the normalization of bodies.

I am not suggesting we declare open season on the sale of babies or on technological intervention into reproduction. Rather, I am suggesting that the incoherencies that plague ethical discourses on issues such as surrogacy would appear to arise from an illegitimate attempt to separate these practices from the everyday social field of power and knowledge which constitutes our desires and capacities. As a consequence of this separation, unconditional opposition to these practices, including that within feminism, is based on at least two spurious assumptions: that the women involved have been duped and coerced into fulfilling the needs of a patriarchal system which exploits women; and that there is a space for the exercise of moral agency outside of and uncontaminated by the norms and values of our social structure.[32] Given that pregnant embodiment is central to the reproduction of our social order, such a stance risks making pregnancy unethical in itself.

Conclusion: bodies, society, ethics

There is much to suggest that women involved in surrogacy and IVF have been neither coerced nor duped (at least no more than the rest of us). And there is much to suggest that surrogacy can be considered a logical extension of a social field that fosters a desire to reproduce, assumes that relations between individuals are based on free and equal contracts, and consists of a network of knowledges and practices which transform bodies as they inform them with meaning and value. It would seem, then, that ethical questions—about which bodies can be altered, by whom, and to what end—need to be directed toward the social field in general rather than to individuals. Immediate concerns about the emotional well-being of surrogates and potential economic exploitation of birth mothers and their children can be simply addressed by not giving the surrogacy contract any legal weight, as the NBCC suggests. Yet such a "solution," necessarily but paradoxically, challenges all our assumptions about individual autonomy, free and equal contracts, and relations of exchange. If pregnant women are to be considered as embodied selves with the same mode of agency as others and at the same time spared the charge of participating in an unethical reproduction of patriarchal social relations, then it is necessary to re-think our model of social relations and its understanding of ethics.

Foucault's account of the social construction of bodies suggests the need to widen the focus of ethics from that which regulates relations between individuals to a critical analysis of the political investments in the knowledges and practices which constitute our embodied being-in-the-world. Such a definition of ethics is not new. It comes from the Greek meaning of "ethos" as one's habitat consisting of the habits that go to make up one's character. Foucault, following this idea, defines "ethos" as a "manner of being" and ethics as a practice, a technique of self-formation.[33] Such a definition of ethics takes into account the contribution biomedical science makes to our embodied being in the world. Not just in highlighting its responsibility for the restoration of the embodied self, but also its complicity in the normalization of bodies, in the ongoing constitution of the habits and capacities that determine our "free" activity.

What Foucault suggests is a need to open up other possibilities for bodies beyond those that make us useful to our economic system. He suggests that "the target nowadays is not to discover what we are, but to refuse what we are. . . . We have to promote new forms of subjectivity through the refusal of this kind of individuality."[34] Using the idea of the body as aesthetic material, he suggests that it is possible to "create ourselves as a work of art."[35] That is, we should create ourselves differently without reference to the normalizing disciplinary structure and without domination and exclusion of others. As Iris Young suggests, following Sally Gadow's reflections on aging and illness, pregnancy can be most constructively viewed as an experience of the body in such an aesthetic mode.[36] This "aesthetics of existence" is not a project of "liberation" from practices such as biomedicine, understood as something that restricts our freedom. Rather, it is a project for enlarging the sphere of positive freedom, as Patton puts it.[37] It is a project for expanding our capacities, working on our bodies to extend the sphere of possibilities of action beyond those that merely feed into the efficiency of our social and economic structure. Insofar as biomedicine may contribute to a restoration of bodily capacities, then, it contributes to an aesthetics of existence. But insofar as it contributes to our objectification, subjection, and normalization, then, it is counterproductive to such an aesthetics.

Notes

I am grateful to Paul Komesaroff, Catriona Mackenzie, Paul Redding, and Philipa Rothfield for their useful comments on an earlier draft of this paper.

1   National Bioethics Consultative Committee, *Surrogacy: Report 1* (Commonwealth of Australia, April, 1990). The NBCC was a national committee formed in 1988 to advise the Australian Government on bioethical issues that might have a bearing on public policy. Its report on surrogacy was prepared by a subcommittee chaired by Max Charlesworth, who is understood to be the principal author. The NBCC was replaced in 1991 by the Australian Health Ethics Committee. All text citations are to this report.

2   Isaiah Berlin, "Two Concepts of Liberty," *Four Essays on Liberty* (Oxford, Oxford University Press, 1969).

3   This has been the case at least since the political theory of John Locke, who claims that "every Man has Property in his own person. . . . The Labour of his Body, and the work of his hands, we may say, are properly his" (*Two Treatises of Government,* ed. P. Laslett [New York, Mentor, 1965], p. 328).

4   For example, Dr. Diana Kirby (Melbourne Feminist Legal Theory Group) argues against surrogacy on the grounds that a surrogate mother cannot predict the strength of her emotional attachment to the child at the time of birth. NBCC, *Surrogacy Report,* p. 17.

5   Daniel Callahan, "Autonomy: A Moral Good, not a Moral Obsession," *Hastings Center Report* (October 1984), p. 42. I am grateful to Deborah Keighley-James for bringing this article to my attention.

6   Roslyn Diprose, "The Surrogacy Contract," in Moira Gatens and Marion Tapper, eds., *Re-reading the Sexual Contract* (Allen and Unwin, forthcoming).

7   Oliver Sacks, *The Man Who Mistook His Wife for a Hat* (London, Picador, 1985).

8   Ibid., pp. 63–66.

9   Drew Leder, *The Absent Body* (Chicago, University of Chicago Press, 1990), 80.

10 See, for example, Martin Heidegger, "Letter on Humanism," in David Farrell Krell, ed., *Martin Heidegger: Basic Writings* (New York, Harper and Row, 1977).

11 See, for example, R. Diprose, "In Excess: The Body and the Habit of Sexual Difference," *Hypatia* 6, no. 3: 156–171, and "A Genethics that Makes Sense," in R. Diprose and R. Ferrell, eds., *Cartographies: Poststructuralism and the Mapping of Bodies and Spaces* (Sydney, Allen and Unwin, 1991).

12 Leder, *Absent Body,* p. 71.

13 Ibid., p. 73.

14 Paul Patton, partly following Berlin, describes the restriction of one's "positive freedom" as an internal (as opposed to external) limitation placed on the agent's capacity to act, in "Taylor and Foucault on Power and Freedom," *Political Studies* 37, no. 2 (1989): 262.

15 David Schenck, "The Texture of Embodiment: Foundation for Medical Ethics," *Human Studies* 9, no. 1 (1986): 46.

16 Ibid., p. 51.

17 Iris M. Young, "Pregnant Embodiment: Subjectivity and Alienation," in *Throwing Like a Girl and Other Essays in Feminist Philosophy and Social Theory* (Bloomington, Indiana University Press, 1990).

18 Merleau-Ponty, for example, argues that habituation, the constitution of one's lived body, involves the nonconscious transfer of habits, gestures, and movements between bodies. This process begins when children mimic the conducts of others. The capacities one develops varies depending on one's cultural situation and personal history. And, presumably one's cultural situation is informed by socially specific discourses and practices which govern what bodies mean and what they can do. See M. Merleau-Ponty, "The Child's Relations with Others," in *The Primacy of Perception,* ed. James Edie (Evanston, Ill., Northwestern University Press, 1964).

19 Michel Foucault, *Discipline and Punish: The Birth of a Prison,* trans. Alan Sheridan (Harmondsworth, Penguin, 1977), p. 27.

20 Foucault, "The Subject and Power," afterword to Hubert L. Dreyfus and Paul Rabinow, *Michel Foucault: Beyond Structuralism and Hermeneutics* (Brighton, Harvester Press, 1982), p. 221.

21 Patton, "Taylor and Foucault," p. 262.

22 Foucault, "Body/Power," in Colin Gordon, ed., *Power/Knowledge: Selected Interviews and Other Writings 1972–1977 by Michel Foucault* (Brighton, Harvester Press, 1980), p. 58.

23 Foucault, "Omnes et Singulatim: Towards a Critique of Critical Reason," *The Tanner Lectures on Human Values*, vol. 2 (Salt Lake City, University of Utah Press, 1981).

24 Foucault, *Discipline and Punish*, p. 25.

25 Foucault, "The Politics of Health in the Eighteenth Century," in *Power/Knowledge*, p. 170.

26 Ibid., p. 172.

27 Foucault, "Subject and Power," p. 121.

28 Foucault, *Discipline and Punish*, p. 212.

29 Ibid., part 3, ch. 1. According to Foucault's analysis, individualization in institutions proceeds through the segmentation of time and space. The time and space segments occupied by individuals are codified and ranked; each has a meaning and value and will incur different degrees of discipline and observation. An individual takes on a social identity according to the code and rank of the space occupied.

30 Foucault, "Politics of Health," p. 174.

31 Moira Gatens, *Feminism and Philosophy: Perspectives on Difference and Equality* (Cambridge, Polity, 1991), pp. 34–44.

32 See, for example, Susan Sherwin's argument against reproductive technology in "Feminist and Medical Ethics: Two Different Approaches to Medical Ethics," *Hypatia* 4, no. 2 (1989), pp. 57–72, and arguments against surrogacy in Meggitt, *Surrogacy: In Whose Interest*.

33 Foucault, "Politics and Ethics: An Interview," in Paul Rabinow, ed., *The Foucault Reader* (Harmondsworth, Penguin, 1984), p. 377, and *The Use of Pleasure*, vol. 2 of the *History of Sexuality*, trans. Robert Hurley (New York, Random House, 1985), pp. 25–32.

34 Foucault, "Subject and Power," p. 216.

35 Foucault, "On the Genealogy of Ethics: An Overview of Work in Progress," in *The Foucault Reader*, p. 346.

36 Young, "Pregnant Embodiment," p. 165, and Sally Gadow, "Body and Self: A Dialectic," *Journal of Medicine and Philosophy* 5 (1980): 172–185.

37 Patton, "Taylor and Foucault," p. 276.

Female bodies and food: a case of ethics and psychiatry

Denise Russell

In the eyes of many of its practitioners, psychiatric medicine is a value neutral inquiry. In this chapter, I attempt to expose the incorrectness of this assumption by focusing on one area, the "eating disorder." I argue that the framework of understanding that flows from psychiatric medicine leads to certain kinds of treatment and to the exclusion of other ways of understanding. The psychiatric medical approach is unsubstantiated. This leads to a moral problem in recommending treatments that do not have a good record of success and to another moral problem in excluding from consideration directions of thought that could lead to a richer understanding.

In North America and some other countries psychiatry has shifted direction within the last decade. Psychoanalysis has lost ground to biological theories, in which mental illnesses or disorders are viewed as biological problems, usually with genetic bases. If these conditions are amenable to cures at all, then, it is "biological cures" that are thought to be appropriate—cures, that is, that alter biochemistry, such as psychiatric medications and electroconvulsive therapy (E.C.T.). This model has been applied to a range of "disorders" that includes schizophrenia, depression, and the eating disorders.

The model, however, is problematic. While its guiding assumption is that the particular mental disorder is a biological fault, there is no consensus on the nature of this fault in any area of psychiatric research; this is in spite of the fact that in some of these areas (such as, for example, the investigation of schizophrenia and depression) research has been going on for decades. Also, the model doesn't just exist in a research vacuum; it extends into the treatment, even when it is acknowledged that the theoretical rationale for treatment is very shaky. The "biological" treatments may, on occasion, give temporary relief, but many of the medications are addictive and hazardous, and E.C.T. is known to cause brain damage. So even in this respect the model is questionable. This whole subject is of particular relevance to women, because women draw on psychiatric services more than men and they are more likely to be diagnosed as schizophrenic, depressed, or suffering from the eating disorders.

Problems in the view of eating disorders taken by biological psychiatry

I will now turn to the "eating disorders." What does medical psychiatry regard as an eating disorder? It acknowledges four main categories: two rare ones that occur in babies, and anorexia nervosa and bulimia nervosa. The diagnostic criteria for these disorders, as specified in the *Diagnostic and Statistical Manual of Mental Disorders*, are as follows:

Diagnostic criteria for anorexia nervosa
a. Refusal to maintain body weight over a minimal normal weight for age and height, e.g., weight loss leading to maintenance of body weight 15% below that expected; or failure to make expected weight gain during period of growth, leading to body weight 15% below that expected.
b. Intense fear of gaining weight or becoming fat, even though underweight.
c. Disturbance in the way in which one's body weight, size, or shape is experienced, e.g., the person claims to "feel fat" even when emaciated, believes that one area of the body is "too fat" even when obviously underweight.
d. In females, absence of at least three consecutive menstrual cycles when otherwise expected to occur ("primary" or "secondary" amenorrhoea.).[1]

Diagnostic criteria for bulimia nervosa
a. Recurrent episodes of binge eating (rapid consumption of a large amount of food in a discrete period of time).
b. A feeling of lack of control over eating behavior during the eating binges.
c. Regular self-induced vomiting, use of laxatives or diuretics, strict dieting or fasting, or vigorous exercise in order to prevent weight gain.
d. An average of at least two binge eating episodes a week for at least three months.
e. Persistent overconcern with body shape and weight.[2]

Some investigators disagree with these criteria—for example, some don't want to include amenorrhoea in the requirements for anorexia nervosa.[3] Nonetheless, all seem to agree that the disorders are much more common in women than in men.

Attempts to isolate the biological fault in eating disorders follows a similar pattern to other areas of psychiatry. Three broad strategies are used, each of which, I shall claim, is faulty. First, there is an appeal to genetics to argue that some people have a genetic disposition to developing anorexia nervosa. I believe that while this may be true, the research to date has not established that conclusion, and even if it did, the conclusion on its own is not enough to support a medical orientation. Second, there is an assumption that the disorders are caused by faulty chemistry and research is carried out in search of various possible chemical faults. The argument I wish to put here is that while there may be certain chemical differences between a person diagnosed with one of these disorders and others, we don't need to conclude that these chemical differences are the cause of the disorder. Third, newer imaging techniques are used to attempt to isolate abnormal brain patterns in those suffering from the disorders. However, even though very interesting correlations might emerge from this approach, these correlations need not tell us anything about causation.

Even if this critique of the medical psychiatric perspective is successful, it could still be argued that the treatments that emerge from it are useful in practice. However, the most common medications for anorexia nervosa, the antidepressants, are not superior to placebos, when tested under double-blind conditions; further, the antischizophrenic drugs, which have also been used, have failed to show any marked benefit in a recent survey.[4] Bulimia nervosa, too, is sometimes treated with antidepressants; as for anorexia nervosa, trials have failed to substantiate any claim to their effectiveness, and a significant number of the deaths that occur in people with eating disorders are the result of overdoses with antidepressants.[5] One particular class of antidepressants, the monamine oxidase inhibitors, has also been used for bulimia nervosa; these drugs can be very dangerous if you take them with certain common foods. It is hard to evaluate their effect in treating bulimia nervosa as most subjects drop out of the tests because of intolerable side effects.[6] In summary, it cannot be argued that the treatment proposals that emerge from the biological model of eating disorders have been justified by their practical usefulness.

Genetic evidence

Let me consider the argument in more detail. First, the genetic evidence. Is there a genetic component to the eating disorders? This question has been studied for anorexia nervosa but not yet for bulimia nervosa. Some studies simply appeal to the finding that there is an increased incidence of anorexia nervosa in family members to argue that there is therefore a genetic component to it.[7] This is, however, a very weak basis on which to assert a genetic influence as it could easily be some aspect of the family social context that causes the disorder in more than one member. There are in fact strong suggestions coming out of the literature to support the view that families containing members with eating disorders give health and fitness an exceptional priority[8] and that they also place greater than average importance on food and eating.[9]

A recent review of twin studies in this area indicates that in about 50 percent of twenty-four pairs of "identical" twins both had anorexia nervosa. Methodological problems, however, lead to skepticism about this result. There is, for instance, a question about whether all the pairs were truly identical.[10] As nonidentical twins share about the same number of genes as ordinary siblings, a finding of concordance for a disorder in nonidentical twins may not tell us anything about genetics. In a recent study that is frequently referred to as "establishing a genetic base for anorexia nervosa," Holland et al. found that nine out of sixteen identical twins shared anorexia nervosa, but for fourteen pairs of nonidentical twins only one pair shared the disorder. This study claims to have sorted out the methodological problems of previous studies by the use of a more precise measure of zygosity to determine whether the twins are identical or not.[11] But there is another methodological problem that the authors fall into; they knew whether the twins were identical or not at the time they made the assessment of whether the person had anorexia. There is therefore the possibility of the well-established problem of experimenter bias here, and it is puzzling why the researchers did not proceed in a way that would avoid it. Also, this study is susceptible to a further criticism that people who look alike tend to be treated alike, which might explain how a disorder might be shared by identical twins quite independently of any genetic mechanisms.

Finally, it may be true that anorexia has a genetic component without it being the case that it should be regarded primarily as a biological disorder. After all, while it may be true that musical ability has a genetic component, we are not tempted to say that this is biologically determined. Thus to agree that there is a genetic aspect to anorexia nervosa does not imply that it is primarily biological in nature.

Body chemistry

The second strand of the argument for the biological model of eating disorders delves into body chemistry. The dominant theory along these lines asserts that the disorders are diseases of the neuroendocrine system.[12] The endocrine system involves hormones that have widespread effects on bodily functions and metabolism. This system is closely linked to the brain, which both influences hormonal patterns and is, in turn, influenced by them; hence we can talk of a "neuroendocrine system." The menstrual cycle is a part of this system. In women with anorexia nervosa, this cycle stops; indeed, those suffering from anorexia nervosa have low levels of the sex hormones.[13] These hormones are under the control of another hormone released by part of the brain called the hypothalamus. It is not possible to measure the hypothalamic hormone directly, but indirect measures show that there are abnormal levels of the hypothalamic hormone in women suffering from anorexia nervosa.[14] The hypothalamus is involved in the control of appetite, satiation, sexuality, and emotion, all of which are changed in anorexia nervosa. Drawing all these strands together, it is argued that anorexia nervosa is a primary disease of the neuroendocrine system, notably of the hypothalamus and the related areas of the brain.[15] A more specific hypothesis claims that there is an increase in the chemical triggers that decrease feeding in anorexia nervosa. There is some evidence for this.[16]

The mere fact of cessation of periods in women with anorexia nervosa forces us to grant that there is a biological change. However, we do not need to accept that the basic problem is biological. Weight and level of nutrition in the diet seem to be the keys to understanding the neuroendocrine changes, because when the weight and nutritional content of the diet are restored to normal, the hormone levels return to normal, too.[17] Weight on its own, however, is not a sufficient explanation, as not all anorexic subjects regain normal endocrine and menstrual function as soon as their weight returns to normal.[18] Nonetheless, these functions do return to normal when the women move off starvation diets and gain weight. Thus it seems most likely that the dietary restraint causes the neuroendocrine changes rather than the other way around.

In bulimia nervosa a rather similar story is emerging. Periods do not cease and weight may remain normal, but in some other respects the neuroendocrinology of bulimia overlaps with anorexia nervosa.[19] It is also thought that the triggers that signal satiety may be set differently from normal, which may prompt binge eating. There is some indirect chemical evidence for this.[20] Further indirect evidence comes from a study which showed that bulimic subjects were less responsive to chemical signals that lead to the termination of meals because they were hungrier at the end of meals than control subjects.[21]

Can we say then that the basic fault in bulimia nervosa is a neuroendocrine one? Although some researchers draw this conclusion,[22] alternative explanations seem more plausible. Some writers claim that weight changes bring about the neuroendocrine changes[23] but this will not account for those suffering from bulimia nervosa who retain normal weight. Schweiger and others[24] have demonstrated that in spite of their weight status, bulimic sufferers are often effectively in a state of starvation and they claim that it is this nutritional deprivation that causes the neuroendocrine changes. A further piece of relevant research is that neuroendocrine disturbances may result from reduced intake of calories, not just in those with eating disorders, but also in normal subjects.[25] Levy, in a study of the neuroendocrine profile of bulimia nervosa, states that the person with bulimia nervosa may be in a "normal weight malnourished state" but suggests that malnourishment needs to be defined in ways other than by weight parameters.[26] If the primary problems are isolated as weight and lack of adequate diet, then we are not forced to posit a biological cause.

A further line of reasoning that tries to pin bulimia nervosa down to a biological fault runs as follows: there is an association between bulimia nervosa and depression. Depression is caused by a biological fault; therefore bulimia is caused by a biological fault.[27] As I show in *Women, Madness and Medicine*, this claim about the cause of depression doesn't stand up under scrutiny, and the style of argument is an example of the "sleight of hand" maneuver—a weak piece of reasoning in one area is used to back weak reasoning in another.

A variant of this theme is put forward by Pope and Hudson, who argue that bulimia is the result of an underlying depression.[28] Nothing beyond correlation is offered in support of this claim, and the mere fact of correlation is too weak to support a causal conclusion. Indeed, it would be surprising if sufferers of bulimia did not experience some depression related to their eating practices, so the causal link may actually be in the opposite direction from that proposed by Pope and Hudson. Other research reports bear on this issue. Laessle et al. draw attention to the fact that depression in bulimia is no more common than in any other psychiatric conditions and that it may follow on from a diet low in carbohydrates.[29]

Structural studies of the brain
I now turn briefly to the third line of evidence for the biological model—that involving computerized imaging of the brain. Using a type of x-ray scanning called computerized tomography (CT), certain structural changes were observed in the brains of subjects with anorexia nervosa (viz., enlargement of the external cerebrospinal fluid spaces and/or a dilatation of the ventricles); also, recent CT studies of bulimic subjects with normal weight have revealed mor-

phological brain alterations similar to those found with anorexic subjects.[30] There is dispute about whether or not these changes can simply be regarded as the effects of starvation.[31] The research is very new and more research with control subjects is needed to clarify the issue. At most, what it reveals to date is that structural brain changes are a biological marker of the eating disorders; it does not help us sort out what is primary in a causal sense.

Historical and cultural variability of the eating disorders

Anorexia nervosa has been known about at least since the seventeenth century.[32] Yet even in the 1970s one of the key workers in the field declared that anorexia was "rare indeed."[33] In 1984 "it was estimated that one in every 200–250 women between the ages of thirteen and twenty-two suffers from anorexia and that anywhere between 12 and 33 percent of college women control their weight through vomiting, diuretics, and laxatives."[34] Ben Tovim et al. assert that "in just a few years bulimia has gone from being virtually unknown to being described as a "major public health problem" and a disorder of "epidemic proportions."[35] Other writers agree.[36]

Perhaps to some extent the incidence of these disorders was hidden before lists of criteria were specifically developed, but that is unlikely to be sufficient explanation of the apparent historical variability. This feature poses obvious problems for a biological medical approach as presumably women's biology has not varied that much or that suddenly.

This historical variability of eating disorders should also be considered in connection with cultural variability. The above statistics referred to Western culture, specifically that of North America and Western Europe. Anorexia is virtually unknown in China or in the Chinese community in Hong Kong, less common in Russia and Eastern Europe, uncommon in Latin American countries, rare in Malaysia, and increasing in Japan[37] and Australia. One generalization that seems to be supported is that where there is a genuine shortage of food these disorders are rare.[38] These cultural variations pose great difficulties for the biological approach; nonetheless, they are usually ignored in writings defending this position.

Why is the biological psychiatric approach flourishing?

With all these weaknesses in the defense of the medical perspective on eating disorders, how can we explain the fact that this approach is gaining ground? Several factors are likely to be important here. First, there is a bid by psychiatry to improve its status within the medical domain—to show that it is scientific after the attacks by Popper and others on its scientific status when it was dominated by psychoanalysis.[39] In brief, Popper argued that psychoanalysis was unscientific because every conceivable observation could be explained in its terms. Nothing would serve as a possible falsification. This, according to Popper, made the view empty. Modern psychiatrists believe that the drive to be scientific will be fostered if they draw on genetic theory, on chemistry, and on computerized imaging.

I have some sympathy with the criticisms of psychoanalysis, and I think they are particularly apt in this area. There is a proliferation of psychoanalytic theories of the eating disorders that don't sit very easily with each other—for example, the view that the eating disorders are caused by an unconscious conflict resulting in a rejection of femininity conflicts with the view that anorexia is an exaggerated striving to achieve femininity.

Waller et al. claim that "anorexia stems from disapproval by parents of their adolescent daughter's sexuality resulting in her defending it by regression to the orality of infantile sexuality."[40] Chernin also believes that:

> At the heart of an eating obsession is a regression to the infantile condition [to fulfil] a need to regain a relationship to the . . . mystery of female being—a mystery conferred inalienably upon women's lives by our ability to create life and food from the female body. . . . It is as if we are trying to remind ourselves, through our obsessive overvaluation of food, that we have been starved of this positive sense of an inherent female creative power on the basis of which we could elaborate a new and meaningful female social identity.[41]

While this focuses on fantasies underlying anorexia nervosa, Hilde Bruch stresses the actual deprivations experienced by those suffering from eating disorders. These deprivations are a result of "abnormal patterns of family interaction"[42] in infancy. The infant's needs are not appropriately met and ego boundary problems arise. This surfaces most clearly in adolescence. She writes of the patient as someone who is not "seen or acknowledged as an individual in her own right, but . . . valued as someone who would make the life and experiences of the parents more satisfying and complete."[43] Caskey puts forward a Jungian account that "anorexics are caught in a relationship to the animus as it is projected onto the father. . . . Anorexia is the result of a peculiar kind of incest which involves a psychic relationship rather than a physical one."[44]

How can these competing accounts be evaluated? The general problems in the assessment of psychoanalytic theories are applicable here, and an evaluation in terms of the success of treatments that emerge from the perspective is difficult to make because of the lack of long-term follow-up studies.[45] Another source of suspicion of the psychoanalytic approach is that one of the main proponents, Hilde Bruch, actually opposes the use of psychoanalytic interpretation in the treatment of anorexia[46] and Selvini-Palazzoli who for years treated anorexic patients with psychoanalysis has abandoned it for a more directive, strategic intervention.[47] Perhaps psychiatry is right in shedding the links to psychoanalysis in its bid to increase its status within medicine. However, that does not mean that the biological psychiatric account of eating disorders needs to be accepted. I will return to this point later.

There are two other possible reasons for the attention given to the biological medical perspective. One is the background influence of the pharmaceutical companies. The pharmaceutical industry is the second most profitable industry in the world, and it is constantly looking for new markets. There are various ways in which it can have an effect on theorizing, for example, by providing funds for research along the lines that support theories that lead into pharmaceutical treatments. I also suspect that there may be some misogyny tied up with the new psychiatric directions. If more women than men suffer from eating disorders, and if the basic problem is one of faulty biology, then this can serve as a justification for according inferior status to these women.

Alternative accounts of the eating disorders

Although my main focus here is a critique of the medical perspective, it is intriguing to ask what a more acceptable account would look like. There are a couple of directions that seem very hopeful, and I would like briefly to indicate what they are. The first arises from the work of Susan Bordo. She views anorexia as a cultural phenomenon linked to the particular situation of women in modern Western culture.[48] It is "a symptom of some of the . . . distresses of our age."[49] The key cultural phenomena that she claims are important in understanding anorexia are:

1. The belief in dualism: the mind/body split. "This is manifested in the anorexic by a battle between the mind or will and appetite or body. . . . In this battle, thinness represents a triumph of the will over the body."[50]
2. The importance placed on control of the body. "The anorexic, typically,

experiences her life and her hungers as being out of control."[51] She feels powerless.

3. The cultural emphasis on the slenderness of women and the denigration of women. This is manifested in anorexia by a disdain for traditional female roles and social limitations and a "deep fear of 'The Female' with all its more nightmarish archetypal associations: voracious hungers and sexual insatiability."[52]

Many aspects of eating disorders fall into place if this account is accepted. In particular, a plausible explanation can be given of the historical and cultural variability in the occurrence of the eating disorders. The rising incidence of these conditions in recent times has paralleled the decreasing estimates of the ideal body weight in Western culture.[53] This ties in with Bordo's third point. The cultural variability mentioned above is also easily accounted for in Bordo's account. The greater the incidence of eating disorders in Western culture could be related to the above three factors, which are not so significant in other cultures.

Bordo does not accept that anorexia is pathological. Eva Szekely goes one step further in her sociocultural account of what she calls the relentless pursuit of thinness. She believes that the practices which have been labeled "eating disorders" do not represent a radical departure from the lives of other women in similar sociohistorical contexts.[54] Hence she rejects the pathological status of anorexia and in fact avoids talking about "anorexia" and "bulimia." The key question then becomes "What in the sociocultural contexts of women's lives has created the possibility and the necessity for women to engage in the relentless pursuit of thinness?" The answer suggested is that the context is one where "appearance is considered to be woman's major asset, where what women are able to do matters far less than what they look like, where people are raised to be never satisfied in the midst of plenty." She points to the pressures on women to be thin in order to obtain and keep a job, and in order to find and keep the "right calibre" of man. Correlatively, "women have been given the message that their efforts in improving and perfecting their bodies would be rewarded by success in both their personal and professional lives."[55] Although it is difficult to escape from this web, one way forward is to see that it does operate and to ask whose interests it serves. It appears to conflict with the interests of the majority of women.

A final problem with the biological psychiatric approach is that it directs our attention away from accounts such as Szekely's, and yet when one bears in mind the historicocultural variability of so-called eating disorders it seems clearly the direction to take. Deflection from this direction by biological psychiatry could well be dangerous given the lives and suffering that are at stake and given the dubious effectiveness of biological cures.

Conclusion

Medical psychiatry does not exist in a value-neutral realm. "Eating disorders" constitute a new field of interest which is illustrative of what has happened in the research and treatment of "schizophrenia," "depression," and "attention deficit disorders." A particular model of understanding is presented, which defines a research direction and a treatment program. When one theory falling under the model is successfully criticized, another is presented. A string of unsubstantiated theories emerges. The treatments are tied into the model—that is, they are biological, in contrast to the specific theories. They can therefore remain the same through the succession of theories.

If it could be demonstrated that the treatments worked, then perhaps there would be no great ethical problem, except that certain other possibly more fruitful research directions that could otherwise have been taken up were foregone. If however the treatments are not shown to be very beneficial and, indeed, to carry significant dangers—as in the case of "eating disorders"—then an ethical problem emerges quite clearly. Also, the fact that other research directions are excluded is not just of academic interest. If Bordo and Szekely are on the right track, they not only provide a way of thinking about "eating disorders" which reveals why the medical psychiatric perspective must fail; they also open up considerations for all women in modern Western culture to help us to understand the covert forms of oppression. In diverting our gaze from these directions, medical psychiatry belies its purported value neutrality and colludes in the maintenance of the subordination of women.

Notes

1   R. L. Spitzer and J. B. Williams, eds., *Diagnostic and Statistical Manual of Mental Disorders,* 3rd ed., rev. (Washington, American Psychiatric Association, 1987), p. 67.

2   Ibid., pp. 68–69.

3   See E. Eckert, "Characteristics of Anorexia Nervosa," in J. Mitchell, ed., *Anorexia Nervosa and Bulimia: Diagnosis and Treatment* (Minneapolis, University of Minnesota Press, 1985), pp. 4–8, and D. J. Ben-Tovim et al., "Bulimia: Symptom and Syndromes in an Urban Population," *Australian and New Zealand Journal of Psychiatry* 23, no. 1 (March 1989): 73–80.

4   J. Treasure, "Psychopharmacological Approaches to Anorexia and Bulimia," in D. Scott, ed., *Anorexia and Bulimia Nervosa* (New York, New York University Press, 1988), p. 128.

5   Ibid., pp. 129–130.

6   Ibid., p. 130, and B. T. Walsh, et al., "Phenelzine vs. Placebo in 50 Patients with Bulimia," *Archives of General Psychiatry* 45, no. 5 (May 1988): 474.

7   Eckert, "Characteristics of Anorexia Nervosa," p. 14.

8   R. L. Palmer, *Anorexia Nervosa,* 2nd ed. (Harmondsworth, Penguin, 1988), 67.

9   Ibid., p. 71.

10 Eckert, "Characteristics of Anorexia Nervosa," p. 14.

11 A. J. Holland, et al., " 'Anorexia Nervosa': A Study of 34 Twin Pairs and One Set of Triplets," *British Journal of Psychiatry* 145 (1984): 414–419.

12 Palmer, *Anorexia Nervosa,* p. 63.

13 Ibid., p. 55.

14 Ibid., p. 57.

15 Ibid., p. 63.

16 Treasure, "Psychopharmacological Approaches," p. 126.

17 Palmer, *Anorexia Nervosa,* p. 57.

18 Ibid., p. 59.

19 A. Levy, "Neuroendocrine Profile of Bulimia Nervosa," *Biological Psychiatry* 25 (1989): 98–109.

20 Treasure, "Psychopharmacological Approaches," p. 126.

21 B. Walch, "Eating Behavior of Women with Bulimia," *Archives of General Psychiatry* 46 (1989): 54–58.

22 Treasure, "Psychopharmacological Approaches," pp. 126–127.

23 P. Garfinkel and D. Garner, *Anorexia Nervosa: A Multi-dimensional Perspective* (New York, Brunnes Mazel, 1982), p. 91.

24 Mentioned in E. Button, "Review of K. M. Pirke et al. eds., *The Psychobiology of Bulimia Nervosa* (Berlin, Springer-Berlag, 1988)," *British Journal of Psychiatry* 154 (April, 1989): 583.

25 Ibid.

26 Levy, "Neuroendocrine Profile," pp. 105–106.

27 Garfinkel and Garner, *Anorexia Nervosa,* p. 91.

28 H. Pope and J. Hudson, *New Hope for Binge Eaters* (New York, Harper and Row, 1985), p. 39.

29 Mentioned in Button, "Review of Pirke," p. 583.

30 J. C. Krieg et al., "Brain Morphology and Regional Cerebral Blood Flow in Anorexia Nervosa," *Biological Psychiatry* 25 (1989): 1041.

31 Ibid., p. 1042; G. W. Hoffman et al., "Cerebral Atrophy in Bulimia," *Biological Psychiatry* (1989): 894.

32 N. Caskey, "Interpreting Anorexia Nervosa," in S. R. Suleiman, ed., *The Female Body in Western Culture* (Cambridge, Harvard University Press, 1986), p. 175.

33 H. Bruch, *Eating Disorders* (New York, Basic Books, 1973), p. 4.

34 S. Bordo, "Anorexia Nervosa: Psychopathology as the Crystallization of Culture," in I. Diamond and L. Quinby, eds., *Feminism and Foucault* (Boston, Northeastern University Press, 1988), p. 88.

35 Ben Tovim et al., "Bulimia," p. 38.

36   Pope and Hudson, *New Hope for Binge Eaters*, p. 38.

37   S. Lee et al., "Anorexia Nervosa in Hong Kong: Why Not More in Chinese?" *British Journal of Psychiatry* 154 (May 1989): 683–688.

38   R. Berkow, ed., *The Merck Manual of Diagnosis and Therapy*, 14th ed. (Rahway, N.J., Merck Sharp and Dohme, 1982), p. 1904.

39   K. Popper, *Conjectures and Refutations* (London, Routledge and Kegan Paul, 1963), pp. 33–50.

40   J. F. Waller et al., "Anorexia Nervosa: A Psychosomatic Entity," in R. M. Kaufman, and M. Heilman, eds., *Evolution of Psychosomatic Concepts* (London, Hogarth Press, 1965).

41   K. Chernin, *The Hungry Self* (New York, Harper and Row, 1985), p. 197.

42   H. Bruch, *The Golden Cage* (New York, Vintage, 1979), 112.

43   Ibid., p. 36.

44   Caskey, "Interpreting Anorexia Nervosa," pp. 185–187.

45   J. Sayers, "Psychodynamic and Feminist Approaches to Anorexia and Bulimia Nervosa," in Scott, *Anorexia Nervosa and Bulimia*, p. 92.

46   Ibid., p. 90.

47   Ibid., p. 92.

48   Bordo, "Anorexia Nervosa," p. 112.

49   Ibid., p. 89.

50   Ibid., p. 95.

51   Ibid., p. 96.

52   Ibid., p. 102.

53   S. L. Bartky, "Foucault, Femininity and the Modernization of Patriarchal Power," in Diamond and Quinby.

54   E. Szekely, *Never Too Thin* (Toronto, Women's Press, 1988), p. 39.

55   Ibid., pp. 18, 182, 190–191.

Glossary

Communitarian. Someone who believes that the establishment or maintenance of community is the chief goal of social and political action.

Discourse. A body of meaning considered as a social and cultural practice within one or more institutional settings. Different discourses are distinguished from each other by their internal structure, their themes, and the social settings within which they occur.

Embodiment. A term used to refer to the conscious lived experience of the body, based on the philosophical view that human experience cannot be properly understood in terms of the activity of consciousness or of thinking abstracted from the body.

Epicureanism. An ethical doctrine, originating in antiquity, that focuses on the importance of friendship in coping with disease or in recuperating from injury.

Epistemology. The theory of knowledge.

Feudal. A decentralized and fragmented form of patrimonial rule associated particularly with the European Middle Ages.

Gendercide. The fear that the use of sex-selection techniques will result in the systematic elimination of female embryos.

Hermeneutics. The theory of interpretation. The term is used in different ways, but often refers to the study of the interpretation of particular texts or, more generally, of configurations of signs able to be considered as texts. Such configurations might include, for example, the experience, context, and meaning of illness.

Language Game. A concept introduced by the philosopher Ludwig Wittgenstein to emphasize the manner in which language and action interpret each other reciprocally. Originally intended to refer to small-scale languages within special spheres, it was expanded to cover parts of existing languages and the ways in which they are employed in discourse.

Lifeworld. In phenomenology, the lived world, or the world of immediate experience.

Metaethics. The study of the nature of ethical thinking and the structure of ethical propositions.

Microethics. The field of moral action within the lifeworld. Microethical events are imbedded in relationships, are determined by contingent local circumstances, and need not be formulated in the terms of conventional moral discourse.

Normative ethics. That part of ethics in which general statements are made about right or desirable conduct.

Ontology. The philosophy of that which exists.

Patriarchy. The rule of the (male) head of household.

Patrimonialism. A system of government organized around a royal, imperial, or aristocratic household.

Phenomenology. A philosophical movement, often associated with the philosopher Edmund Husserl, which bases philosophical reflection on descriptions of ordinary conscious experience. A variety of phenomenological methods has been developed; the focus of the descriptions may include perceptions, cognition, affective and evaluative processes, experiences of the body, and so on.

Postmodernism. A diverse cluster of theories and theoretical perspectives in philosophy, cultural theory, art, and architecture with the common theme of a profound skepticism toward the moral, cultural, and philosophical ideals of modernity, the Enlightenment, and liberal democracy. The term is used in widely different ways, and there is much debate about its theoretical status; it may therefore be better regarded as an intellectual climate rather than as a coherent movement.

Pro-natalism. A cultural attitude influencing women to think that they can be "real" women only if they have children.

Rational Asceticism. The methodical and economical organization of social action and life conduct.

Reproductive Technology. A variety of techniques of assisted procreation which include in vitro fertilization and other methods for facilitating the creation of human embryos and their transfer into women.

Republicanism. A view of the world that emphasizes the importance of public things and public action.

Romanticism. A view of the world that focuses on the plasticity, change, intensification, and dissolution of bodily states and on the transgression of bodily limits.

Stoicism. An ethical doctrine, originating in antiquity, that emphasizes the importance of fortitude and courage in dealing with bodily pain and injury.

Index

Notes on Contributors

Alison Caddick is a social worker currently completing her Ph.D. in the department of history and philosophy of science at the University of Melbourne. She is an editor of *Arena Magazine*.

Max Charlesworth is professor emeritus of philosophy at Deakin University, Victoria, and well known for his work in the field of ethics.

Rosalyn Diprose lectures in philosophy at the University of New South Wales. She is coeditor, with Robyn Ferrell, of *Cartographies: Poststructuralism and the Mapping of Bodies and Spaces* (Allen and Unwin, 1991) and author of *The Bodies of Women: Ethics, Embodiment and Sexual Difference* (Routledge, 1994).

Paul A. Komesaroff is a physician, medical researcher, and philosopher at the Baker Medical Research Institute, Melbourne, where he is executive director of the Eleanor Shaw Centre for the Study of Medicine, Society and Law.

Catriona Mackenzie is a lecturer in philosophy at Macquarie University, where she teaches courses in moral philosophy, feminist philosophy, and applied ethics. Her interests include feminist philosophy, bioethics, moral psychology, and aspects of contemporary French philosophy. She is currently working on a book on the concept of bodily autonomy and its application to biomedical ethics.

Peter Murphy is senior lecturer in politics at the University of Ballarat and editor of *Thesis 11*.

Paul Redding is a medical practitioner and lecturer in philosophy at the University of Sydney.

Philipa Rothfield is a lecturer in philosophy at La Trobe University. She has published on the body, feminism and social theory, postmodernism epistemology, and psychoanalysis. She is currently writing a book on the moving body.

Denise Russell is a senior lecturer in the department of general philosophy at the University of Sydney. She has worked for many years in groups promoting alternatives to medical psychiatry and reform of the mental health law. In late 1994 she published a book entitled *Women, Madness and Medicine*.

Doug White is dean of education at La Trobe University and an editor of *Arena Journal*.

Library of Congress Cataloging-in-Publication Data
Troubled bodies : critical perspectives on postmodernism, medical
ethics, and the body / edited by Paul A. Komesaroff.
Includes index.
ISBN 0-8223-1676-5 (alk. paper). — ISBN 0-8223-1688-9 (pbk. :
alk. paper)
1. Medical ethics.   2. Feminist theory.   3. Postmodernism.
I. Komesaroff, Paul A.
R724.T68   1995
174'.2—dc20   95-16274CIP